BODYSHAPING
for the Over 30s

BODYSHAPING
for the Over 30s

A Balanced Guide to
Shape Where You Want It

By Ros Cruickshank
L.C.S.P. Phys.

foulsham
LONDON • NEW YORK • TORONTO • SYDNEY

foulsham
Yeovil Road, Slough, Berkshire, SL1 4JH

ISBN 0-572-01532-1

Phototypeset in Great Britain by Typesetting Solutions, Slough, England.
Printed in Great Britain by Cox & Wyman Ltd, Reading.

To Jack Read

Acknowledgements

I very much wish to thank the following people for all their kind help, interest and support:

Daphne Bishop, Elsa Edwards, Barbara Harman, Wendy Henderson, Pat Ireland, Judy and Robin Little, Ron Mann, Mary Miles, Dr Tony Palframan, Debbie Ross, Terry Stacey, Glenn Thorpe; and Sue Richardson for her invaluable help with the proof-reading.

Contents

Introduction

Do you want to do away with those extra inches from all the wrong places – to shape up and tone up?

Every woman is conscious of her body. It's too fat, too thin, too short, too tall, ugly, pretty, old, young, moves effortlessly or creaks along. You feed it, clothe it; you are pleased with it or dissatisfied.

You are conscious of its SHAPE.

Bodyshaping is about how to shape your body if you are not 100 per cent thrilled with what you've got; and if you know you are not totally healthy or fit, to help you do something about it. The craze for keeping fit and being bone-thin may pass, but women through the ages have always been concerned about their shape and the problem of getting into, and looking good in, their clothes.

The combination of a new eating pattern and daily exercises with, if it appeals to you, a safe work-out in a multi-gym is the perfect way to achieve this. But if your approach is haphazard, half-hearted, fanatical or extreme this will be reflected in the results. You may not even be successful. An understanding of yourself and a balanced, safe approach is vital, so think about why you need to shape up. Overweight, extra inches, fluid retention or a sluggish system may have a more subtle root cause than simply not taking enough exercise. Tiredness, stress, loneliness, boredom, tension, depression and, of course, pain can all be responsible for keeping you in poor shape. The expressions 'comfort eating' and 'cupboard love' did not originate for nothing! On the other hand, bad eating habits may be the cause of your tiredness or depression.

Who will read this book?

Bodyshaping is principally for women over 30, when 'middle age spread' becomes a threat, but the 'problems' or attitudes mentioned above apply to a very large proportion of women regardless of age. You may be a girl of about 16 or within the age range too often deprecatingly referred to as 'middle age'. The exercises and diets offered here cannot be applied only to the young or only to the older woman because they are *balanced*, therefore their benefits can be enjoyed by everyone. What *is* important is your understanding and approach to your system. You can be healthy, energetic, lively, supple and mobile at 16, 36 and 66! Or at any of these ages you can be the opposite – experiencing poor health, a sluggish metabolism, stress, indulging in comfort eating or feeling half-dead most days. You probably know that you are not only stiffening up but also are not as actively able as you would like to be or used to be.

Whatever your age, you must consider first your overall state of health. If the way you feel is attributable to a medical condition of any kind you must talk with your doctor before you exercise or diet; you may have to accept his or her decision that you should not diet, slim, or exercise specifically in order to shape.

If, on the other hand, you enjoy excellent health, vigour and mobility, regardless of your age, you can slim-diet more boldly and exercise more actively; in other words, make a greater demand upon yourself. Most people will fall between these two extremes, so if you are older or out of condition, be realistic. Make sure that you are in the excellent health that you think you are. It has been known for the result of a medical check-up to surprise, distressfully, the most healthy-seeming person. If you are suffering from a sluggish metabolism, depression, fatigue, lack of confidence, then your approach should be gentler and slower. This is where you must be really honest and not kid yourself that you are in the first category when really you are in the second! The aim is the same. So it is a question of the correct approach and maybe a little longer time to achieve it.

However, these principles are not for you if you are actually disabled in any way, with a physical or mental handicap. You will require nutrition and exercise routines to suit you at a different specialised level.

Bodyshaping should be particularly successful if you are daunted by the thought of rigorous exercise routines and dietary disciplines because nothing of that sort is included here. Strenuous routines are fanatical and extreme and not advisable for any human body. The emphasis throughout *Bodyshaping* is on balance, safety, and qualified and experienced instruction. You will take responsibility for working within your own capabilities, gently increasing these capabilities to achieve your own success story.

So first you must take a long, hard look at yourself! Not only in the mirror, but also at the kind of person you are so that you can make the right decision on the best approach for *you*.

How do you set about it?

Bodyshaping is only possible if you are careful about your diet and your exercise routines.

To slim away those inches requires wise and disciplined eating, and there are one or two ways of doing this without having to try diet after diet.

To tone and re-shape yourself requires specific exercising, otherwise inches fall off in the wrong places and muscles are built up where you least want them.

Exercising in a multi-gym is the most effective way to shape. Look at Mr Universe! He is proof. Of course you won't want to look like him; but if you use the gym equipment correctly you will shape where you want to.

So if you have been fascinated by the thought of exercise equipment and put off by seeing sweaty males straining against enormous weights, rest assured. There is a considerable difference between the way men use the equipment, in order to body-*build*, and the way you will use it, to *shape* yourself.

Where do you find a multi-gym? *Bodyshaping* helps to do this in a later chapter.

Should you use a multi-gym without instruction? The answer is – NO. Much of the equipment is weighted to provide the resistance against which you exercise not only your muscles and joints but also your heart and lungs. Strain any of these and you could suffer an injury, possibly a serious one. You must never pit yourself against the weights but learn how to adapt the equipment to you. *You* must always be the one in control.

Where exercise is concerned, some people have a natural capacity for considerable strength, some by nature have a lesser strength. Some work fast, some slowly. Some like force, others respond better to gentleness. Some equipment is intended more for men than women and all of it is designed for specific parts of your body. You have to be selective. There is also a reasoned order in using weights equipment. It should not be used without a free-standing warm-up first (very effective in itself) and a relaxation afterwards (everyone loves that!). Instruction is essential, and it is given to you here in *Bodyshaping* in simple detail.

If you have anything medically or structurally wrong with you, you *must* consult your doctor first. In certain conditions, like pregnancy, you should not use a multi-gym at all. Precautions and contra-indications are set out later.

To be this self-responsible, you must not ask the impossible of yourself, since everyone has a natural limitation and your body is designed to go only so far. It is interesting to understand a little about how your body works (after all, it is *your* body that you are working out), how it is structured (anatomy) and how it functions (physiology). In *Bodyshaping*, some of the major systems of your body that are involved when you shape and slim are clearly explained, with explanatory diagrams. You will learn a lot about your body and how it works. Did you know, for example, that if all your blood capillaries were put end to end they would stretch round the equator twice? You will find you are a miracle of creation!

You should know a little about food, too, since you cannot manage without it for long. The literature available on nutrition and calorie-counts is overwhelming. *Bodyshaping* tells you simply and clearly why you eat, what to eat, where to find it and how to balance your overall diet. The idea is to give you enough information, not to swamp you with irrelevant facts which put you off. After all, it is not so long ago that much of the knowledge we have today was unknown even by scientists and nutritionists, let alone the general public. Yet people, if their diet was balanced, were just as healthy. It is too easy nowadays to be blinded by science and to make such a meal out of eating!

Bodyshaping shows you how to eat well and sensibly. It also gives you five slimming diets: all balanced, safe and effective. Which suits you? See your doctor first if you are not sure. Extremes of diet can be as harmful as fanatical exercising but these diets are all balanced and will help you to lose weight if you keep to the instructions. *All* slimming diets require self-discipline and self-control. Good intentions and passionate motivation alone are not enough. But this book helps you to help yourself, with a variety of factual and psychological approaches which are sensible and effective, and fun too.

Many of your questions on exercising are at last answered here, too. For example, 'Why should I exercise at all?', 'What is aerobics?' and 'Why do exercise and diet go together?' You are given clear instructions on how you should go about your new exercise routines. The warm-up is a sequence of movements designed to affect every part of you: to mobilise you, keep you supple, improve your circulation and breathing and wake up a sluggish system. It is very effective on its own to slim, tone and shape you. You can do the warm-up sequence at home, every day, following the illustrations which provide an easy, visual reference as you exercise. If you feel inclined to go along to your local multi-gym, you can follow the *Bodyshaping* gym routine. This is designed especially for women. It is the most effective way to shape, and your results will be quicker than doing the warm-up sequence only. Again, you have detailed instructions on how, why and when (and when not) to do these exercises, with the rules of safety clearly set out.

Effective breathing, relaxation and sleep are vitally important. Don't overlook or be sceptical of 'old wives' tales': there is a reason for putting red flannel around your sore throat and for licking your wounds (if you can reach them!) rather than putting on medication from a bottle. The A-Z of tips and hints (pages 150-91) is compiled from many years of experience, research and observation. It could be much longer!

Bodyshaping is neither a new approach nor yet another fad. These come and go only to be replaced by the next one. Underlying all of them is woman's eternal cry about her shape. This book explains the commonsense way of achieving a good shape: you must tune in with your body's natural functioning, not oppose it, be compatible and complementary with nature, since you are part of nature. Sometimes we fail to see the obvious or don't have the knowledge or courage to do things simply, nature's way. Try it with me and you'll see that it works.

Chapter 1

You can do it: SUCCESS STORIES

*T*here is nothing like a good incentive to set you on the right road to shaping up. Forget the image makers with fancy leotards and time to spare, here are some examples of real people who followed the *Bodyshaping* system and really improved their shape and their health.

About 200 women aged between 16 and 65 attended a series of specialised courses once a week over a four, five or six week period. The classes were held in gyms at local leisure centres. Day classes were attended by women with either school-age children or younger children they had placed into the crèche provided by the centres; married women who did not go out to work; older, retired women; and women who were out of work. Some came alone, some as pairs or groups of friends, some as mother and daughter (and in the last instance it was often the mother who was giving encouragement and confidence to her daughter who perhaps was shy or had a particular problem). Evening classes were usually held early in the evening so that those attending could come straight from work. The evening classes lasted for an hour and the daytime ones for an hour and a half. They were always oversubscribed.

Each session started with a brief period explaining, with large diagrammatical wall-charts, how the body is structured and how it functions, with the emphasis on the skeletal frame and the joints and muscles, in other words the parts of your body that you actively and positively exercise. This was followed by the warm-up sequence to promote suppleness and mobility, to tone muscles, to encourage slimming and weight loss; and to limber-in before using the gym. The classes then learned about the equipment in the multi-gym, how to use it and the benefits of using it for shaping your body. The gyms and other rooms used were all booked in advance for each course so that the classes had private, undisturbed use, especially of the gym. This gave the students the confidence to go on to enter and use the multi-gym where other people, including men, were already using the equipment.

The results of a short course like this, during which many of the aspects of this book were covered, were extremely encouraging and the source of great delight to those involved.

● Several women completely did away with low back pain which had bothered them for a considerable time; some had previously been paying frequent visits to their GPs for help.

● Many said their muscles were toning up 'nicely' and they were beginning to re-shape where they wanted!

● One woman lost one stone in four weeks! This dramatic loss was achieved with no alteration in her diet. She did the warm-up sequence each day at home and the gym routine only once a week at class. Her previously sluggish metabolism 'woke up' and she lost weight, inches, toned up and re-shaped. She felt very well, as did many other women who achieved similar results but over a longer period, with or without dieting.

● Several women toned up their abdominal muscles and at last got rid of their post-baby tummies after trying unsuccessfully for years.

● Several older women noticed that their menopause difficulties diminished: their systems became regulated because they were becoming better balanced and more active overall due to the gentle, frequent exercising which affected all parts of their body. Depression, headaches and other symptoms of the menopause eased and their spirits lifted most enjoyably and rewardingly.

● Colds went: they were 'sweated out' in the gym by those exercising a little more demandingly, following the warm-up sequence and gym routine explained in this book.

● Several women generally cheered up! They found themselves happier and able to take a more objective approach to life. Some felt comforted that they were not the only one experiencing their mood of the moment, whether that moment was temporary or more long-term than they felt able to cope with.

● All were pleased to have instruction on a *balanced* way of living, with safe, sensible exercising, diet and slimming. Only those who had trained as nurses or in a parallel profession had any knowledge of how their bodies worked together with understanding of the damage that can be caused by incorrect exercising and eating habits. All appreciated being able to go to supervised and qualified instruction classes, as they learned and practised, before going on to work more on their own at home or in the gym.

● Most women found that as their breathing improved, their lung capacity increased and their muscles toned up they could walk longer distances without tiring, and going upstairs or up hills became *effortless*.

● Several women found a confidence that they had always lacked. They stopped feeling inferior. Their outlook changed.

● Many experienced a marked improvement in their circulation, as they toned and slimmed, because they could move more easily. They no longer had cold feet or hands.

● The classes also provided a time of fun and laughter for many women who either spent a lot of time on their own for one reason or another or who spent much of their time with small children.

● Many women felt able to bring their individual problems, whether physical or emotional, even domestic difficulties, to the instructor just because she herself was a woman. Many women didn't want, or feel it necessary, to go to a counsellor but here they found the outlet and assistance they needed, together with the extrovert physical activity and participation of the group class, which created a good, healthy balance.

● Once their aims were achieved in the way of losing weight, slimming and toning up – or were well on the way to achievement – many women found that all that was required was a regular exercising at home without the use of the gym. At a later date, when they realised their bodies were getting sluggish again or their muscles were losing tone because they had stopped exercising, all they had to do was the warm-up sequence each day for an amazingly short period (say about a week, or even less) for them to feel the benefits becoming effective and subsequently they felt fitter, more able and generally brighter in outlook.

Chapter 2

Your body: How it WORKS

*B*efore you embark on any course of diet or exercise, it is important to have a basic understanding of your body structures and how the various systems interact, to help you see how good nutrition and regular exercise can help the whole body.

Your skeleton and joints – *the framework*

The first system to consider is your basic bone structure, because your skeleton acts as a supporting and protective framework for everything else. It offers points of fixation for your muscles; and three bony cavities protect delicate internal organs (skull: brain; thorax: heart and lungs; pelvis: reproductive and some of the intestinal organs and the bladder). A baby is born with 214 bones, each designed for a special purpose. Those at the base of the spine fuse during childhood and by puberty the young adult has 207 bones. The five bones in the sacrum have joined together and the four bones in the coccyx have become one, lessening the flexibility of the base of the spine but providing a much more stable, strong and protective cavity for the precious organs within.

When bones connect, or articulate with each other, they form a joint. For the purpose of movement the joints are bound together by ligaments and muscles. These strong ligaments stabilise the joints, keeping the articulating bones in their correct position and allowing movement only in a predetermined, controlled and limited direction.

When physically exercising, you are interested not so much in the comparatively immovable joints like those of your skull and pelvis but the movable ones. Of the

---

The diagram opposite shows how the human skeleton forms the framework for the rest of your body. It is your muscles and fat that create your silhouette or shape.

Joints

A ball and socket joint (1), like those in your shoulder and hip, has a wide range of movement, especially at the shoulder. The arm can move backwards and forwards, up to the side of your head and down again, rotate at the shoulder and swing in a circle. This enormous range of movement is possible because there are very few ligaments at the shoulder joint to stabilise it and limit its movement. It can therefore dislocate more easily than more restricted joints.

A hinge joint (2), like those in your fingers, toes and elbow, can only bend and straighten, like a door hinge moving in only one direction and back.

A pivot joint (3), like that at the top of your neck, has a rotary movement, one bone moving on another in one direction and then back again. The first vertebra, the *atlas*, sits on the second vertebra, the *axis*, enabling your head to turn from side to side.

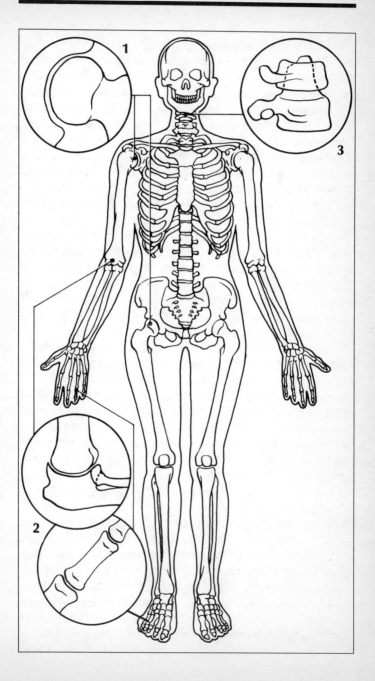

several types of joint, two common ones are: ball and socket joint (such as the shoulder and the hip) and hinge joint (such as the elbow, toes and fingers). Ball and socket construction produces a very wide range of movement but makes the joint less stable and more liable to dislocation. A hinge joint moves like a door hinge, in one direction only, and back.

Force a joint beyond its natural limit (and this can happen if you do not exercise carefully) and the ligaments become wrenched, sprain may occur, the muscles attached may be overstrained and the joint may even dislocate.

As blood passes through your muscles it takes waste matter with it for elimination. This waste matter is fluid and heavy and if your circulation is poor it gravitates to the nearest joint, crystallises and produces stiffness initially. If the crystals are not eliminated, they will become an obstruction to the movement of that joint and a possible forerunner of arthritis.

Apart from the fact that exercise helps to pump blood through your working muscles, preventing waste matter from settling, a specifically designed warm-up and exercise routine takes tension or general stiffness out of your joints, with a noticeably pleasing effect on your everyday activities such as walking, climbing the stairs – even breathing – and giving you a much improved sense of well-being.

Your muscles – *power and movement*

There are three types of muscle: cardiac muscle, which shapes your heart; involuntary muscle which governs bodily functions such as breathing (which is normally an involuntary reflex action) and digestion, over which you have no control; and voluntary muscle which works in obedience to your will. *Bodyshaping* is concerned with voluntary muscle.

The longest muscle in your body runs from the front of your hip to the inside of your knee, passing over two

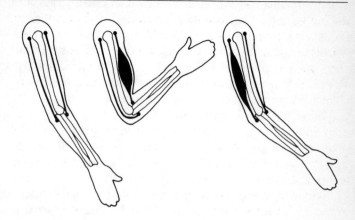

When your arm is straight, the hinge joint at the elbow is open, or extended. When the muscle in front of the elbow joint, the biceps, contracts, the joint closes, or flexes, and the forearm is pulled towards the upper arm, bending the elbow. When the muscle at the back of the joint, the triceps, contracts, the elbow straightens again.

joints. This is *sartorius* and when in action it enables you to sit cross-legged. The shortest muscle is by your upper lip and raises the corners of your mouth when you smile.

Muscles provide the power needed to move the bones forming a joint. For a joint to operate, muscles must be attached at one end to one of the articulating bones, pass over the joint and be attached at the other end to the other articulating bone. They produce the movement by contracting, that is shortening and thickening, when in action, and then relaxing. They do not stretch like elastic! They work in pairs and groups, pulling rhythmically against each other to produce balance, up and down your body, from side to side and from front to back. Even when you are merely standing still, your muscles are constantly at work finely adjusting and readjusting so that you don't fall down by the pull of gravity. They also work to fulfil a deliberate action, such as raising a glass to your lips or tying a bow, so that the movement is controlled precisely as you intend.

A joint will move through its full range only if the muscles are in good condition and tone to produce the required power; there is no impediment obstructing it; and *all* the muscles are functioning to produce the required balance and stability.

If a muscle or group of muscles is not working completely effectively, for whatever reason, imbalance and instability occur and you might fall over (or spill your drink!). Weakness in one area may call for compensation somewhere else, and over a period of time the compensating area becomes affected and the imbalance spreads. For example, if you sprain your right knee joint, or strain the muscles that operate it, the left knee may have to work differently to compensate. If the problem in the right knee persists over a long period of time the left knee may become overworked and you will then have a double problem. As your knee joints are particularly important, because they are essential for bearing your body weight especially whilst you are moving, your general ability to get around will be affected in due course.

The diagram opposite shows the superficial muscles which help to shape you. All work posturally to keep you upright against the pull of gravity, and powerfully when you exercise. According to their size and condition, your silhouette or shape will alter.

1 Sterno-cleido-mastoid	10 Tibialis anterior
2 Deltoid	11 Trapezius
3 Pectoralis major	12 Triceps
4 Biceps	13 Latissimus dorsi
5 Serratus anterior	14 External oblique
6 External oblique	15 Gluteus maximus
7 Rectus abdominus	16 Hamstrings
8 Sartorius	17 Gastrocnemius
9 Quadriceps	18 Achilles tendon

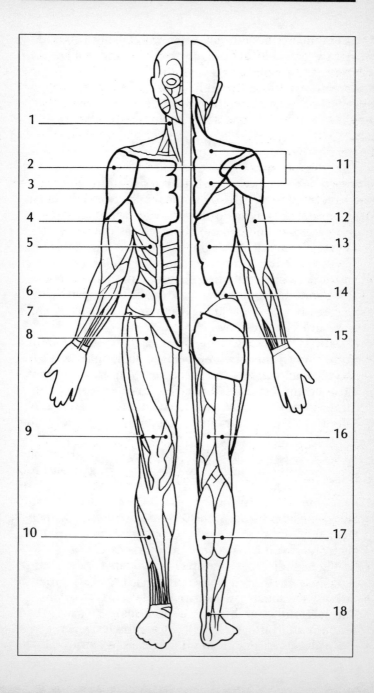

The better the tone of your muscles the better they operate and fulfil your daily activities. Daily exercise of the right kind maintains or improves this tone, affecting your flexibility, agility and shape.

Your muscles – *how they work*

Under a microscope, muscles look rather like those heavy duty cables that contain smaller wires. They are made up of bundles of long fibres, which are in turn composed of bundles of smaller fibres called fibrils.

When a muscle is working, about one-third of its total fibres are active. As they tire, another one-third contract into operation and when they tire the final one-third work and then tire. By this time the first group are rested and ready to work again. This cycle repeats itself while your muscles are active.

Muscle fatigue sets in when each one-third is not sufficiently rested before being called upon again to work. The whole muscle becomes more and more fatigued until it ceases to be able to operate at all, goes into spasm to protect itself and literally brings you to a standstill. This is your muscle's natural way of protecting both itself and you: it is trying to tell you something!

Muscle fatigue can be caused by several factors: exercising the muscle for too long, working against too hard a resistance or carrying too heavy a load. An example of the first situation is when you walk or run for too great a distance. For the second, if you wrench open a very stiff door or window or move heavy furniture. Thirdly, if you carry a very heavy suitcase.

These individual examples are related to the more specific areas of your body that you are using in order to achieve a result. But what happens if you rock-start the car unsuccessfully, grab up your too-heavy suitcase, then run for the bus? How will your muscles react if you offload bags of cement and hump them, all Sunday long, to the far end of your garden where the patio has to be layed before dark, or the rain, or Monday?

The whole of your body is involved in these activities, and the effort is not only considerable but has reached an unwise level. The distress is no longer confined to your muscles but spreads to your heart, lungs and mind. Should you also be overworked during the week, or short of sleep, or have a hang-over, or have just had a row with your family, or be recuperating from a bout of 'flu the ability of your whole system, including your muscles, to work efficiently and effectively is considerably lessened. You know the phrase 'flogging a dead horse'; and can see why it died!

Similar localised stress can occur when exercising in a gymnasium, leading to overall physical and mental distress, if you don't know how, when or why to use the equipment.

Your muscles – *how they shape you*

If you look at the diagram of the skeleton, which is your basic frame, and at the silhouette of your body which is provided by your muscles, especially the superficial muscles and, of course, fat, you see how your body *shape* is formed.

Your skeletal shape is something you cannot alter – it is genetic; and it is a fact that large skeletal frames usually weigh more than small skeletal frames. Your silhouette shape can be altered, but slimming by eating less is often not enough on its own. It's one thing to be thinner, but you may lose inches in the wrong places. And a slimmer shape isn't necessarily any more pleasing to look at. If there is no tone in the muscles they may sag or go wrinkly or stringy!

But it is reassuring to know that if you put a tape measure around a group of muscles in poor tone, for example the top of your thigh, it will measure less a few days or weeks later when correct exercising has begun to tone and 'tighten up' the area, even though you haven't eaten less (providing you haven't eaten more!).

At the other extreme, too much exercising will produce muscle building and the tape measurement will increase! For example, a waitress who works all day, every day, carrying trays of food and piles of dirty dishes can overdevelop the biceps muscles in her upper arms because she is using them so much (although they should be in excellent tone).

On the other hand, if you sit at a desk each day from nine to five you will get a 'spread bottom' by nature of your occupation which does not allow much action of your gluteal muscles (the big muscles in your buttocks). These muscles are very important in maintaining your upright position when standing or walking, two activities which you are not doing much of during the day – and possibly not during the evening either if you like watching TV!

Another major area of muscle which is affected by your general level of exercise is the abdominal muscles. It is an area of the body which is sometimes difficult to tone, especially if you are older, or have borne children and neglected yourself in that area. Your abdomen is a major cavity of your body which contains the viscera: the soft organs of your stomach, liver, gall bladder, pancreas, spleen, kidneys and small and large intestines. These are protected almost entirely by the four large abdominal muscles which are intricately related with each other, reaching from the spine at the back right round to the front, and from your pelvis and hips up to your lower ribs. These muscles are well named 'the abdominal corset'. If they are in poor condition with no tone, they sag and bulge and the soft organs within become displaced by gravity because there is neither a bony structure nor well-toned muscles to prevent this. If you can improve the muscle tone, you will feel, function and look better.

So when you are thinking about the task of shaping yourself, you have to consider how much can be achieved if your occupation is not conducive to either losing inches or changing your shape.

Trying to counteract your sedentary job by spending an hour immediately after work going to an aerobic class or jogging is going from one extreme to the other – and extremes are often not safe. It is the steady, ongoing, moderation-in-all-things approach – both in exercise and eating habits – that achieves results and achieves them permanently.

Circulation – *the merry-go-round*

Blood flows around your body all the time: it is your chief transport system. It is a semi-fluid tissue made up of a yellowy fluid called plasma which contains many substances including water, waste matter, salts, gases, hormones, red and white blood cells and platelets.

The red cells (erythrocytes) give blood its red colour and are responsible for carrying oxygen and nutrients to all your body tissues and taking up waste products, and for distributing heat through your body.

The white cells (leucocytes) wander through your bloodstream, searching for germs and destroying them. They manufacture antibodies which confer immunity to disease.

Platelets (thrombocytes) assist in the clotting of blood. If you cut yourself badly it is the function of the platelets to gather round the wound to prevent you from bleeding to death.

In the process of circulation, oxygenated blood is pumped from the left side of your heart along the vessels (arteries) which diminish in size until they become a network of miniscule arterial capillaries. At this stage all the oxygen, dissolved food and mineral salts pass through the capillary walls into your body cells and waste material is picked up; the now de-oxygenated blood is taken up by another network, venous capillaries, which increase in size, becoming veins to return the blood to your heart. From there it passes to your lungs to be re-oxygenated and then goes back to the heart to be pumped around your body again in a continuous cycle. Depending on your size, you have about 5 litres/7¾ pints of blood in your body.

Exercise assists your circulation, maintaining or increasing your good health and often helping to wake-up a sluggish system. Excessive or unwise exercise, especially if taken by someone medically unwell, can exacerbate a problem. If you are not sure, you must see your doctor before embarking on any unaccustomed physical routine, even if you don't intend it to be strenuous or excessively demanding.

Lymphatics – *one-way system*

Your lymphatic system is a one-way system, moving in the same direction as the blood in your veins, that is, back to your heart.

One of the components of blood is plasma, some of which seeps through your blood capillaries into your tissues and in its new form is called lymph. It picks up bacteria and is absorbed into your lymph capillaries and then carried via lymph vessels to bundles of lymph glands.These filter the bacteria to prevent them being carried on. In this way infections in your body are checked. These glands are situated in specific groups, for example, at your knees and elbows, under your armpits, near your groin, within your abdomen and down the front and sides of your neck. Sometimes when you have an infection these areas are noticeably swollen and tender.

The lymph vessels connect with your bloodstream at points just below your collar bone. Here the lymph flows into the venous return which is about to pass into your heart and on into your lungs.

Along the length of your circulatory and lymphatic systems the veins and lymph vessels all have small valves which prevent 'backwash'.

Respiration – *from the cradle to the grave*

Respiration is an involuntary process which starts at the moment of your birth and continues throughout your life. Air is taken into your lungs where the oxygen is transferred to your blood and travels through your blood stream to every cell in your body, where it is necessary to 'burn up' nutrients and release energy. Carbon dioxide, a waste product of this process, is taken back through the blood stream to the lungs where, with other unwanted products, it is expelled.

Your lungs lie inside your thorax, protected by the bony rib cage. A great many muscles are involved in the production of the respiratory movements. For the purposes of *Bodyshaping* let us consider the intercostal muscles, between the ribs, and the diaphragm, a large dome-shaped muscle below the lungs. The diaphragm descends and flattens when it contracts while the intercostals expand the ribs. The chest space and lungs are thus enlarged, the pressure of the lungs is reduced and air is sucked into them through your nose or mouth. The air passes down your windpipe, or trachea, through two tubes called bronchi (one bronchus to each lung) and into a network of tiny tubes into the air chambers of your lungs.

As the blood passes through the lungs, it picks up this fresh oxygen and deposits the carbon dioxide returned from the cells of the body.

When all the respiratory muscles relax, the diaphragm

rises and the bony cavity formed by the rib cage returns to its original position. Air is forced out, expelling carbon dioxide, excess heat and moisture.

The benefit of breathing through your nose rather than your mouth is that your nose is lined with tiny hairs, or cilia, and with membranes which secrete mucus. The air is warmed as it enters your nostrils so that it is closer to your internal body temperature and it is also filtered by the cilia. Foreign particles such as dust stick to the mucus and you get rid of them when you blow your nose or sneeze. The cilia also move in a wave-like motion to push excess mucus towards your throat where it can be swallowed or spat out to prevent it from passing down into your lungs.

The better the performance of your lungs and heart, the better the performance of the rest of your body and the greater your ability to exercise. When you do exercise, whatever your ability, the performance of your heart and lungs will improve, providing a benefit to your general health. Since your body will require additional oxygen while exercising, the first exercises you should do, those in the warm-up sequence, are designed to prepare your body for the greater demand you will put on it during the gym routine. The first exercise with the equipment is designed especially to limber up your rib cage, and therefore exercise and prepare your lungs ready for the ensuing physical demand.

Digestion – *fuelling the system*

Digestion starts the moment you put food into your mouth. So much emphasis is put on the cosmetic appearance of our teeth that it is easy to forget why we

The digestive system (shown opposite) stretches about 7.5-9 metres/25-30 feet from mouth to anus.

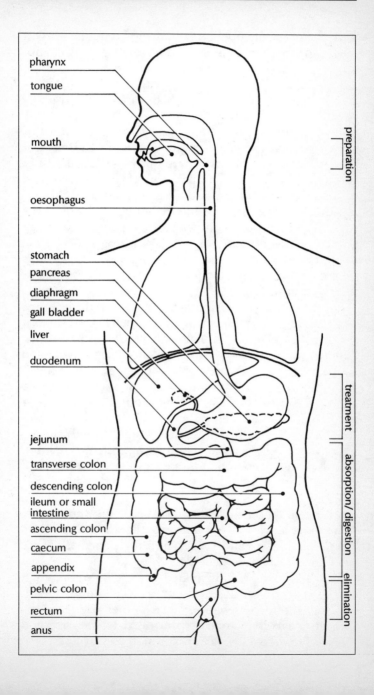

have them! Their function is to chew food and break it down, so that the saliva secreted from the glands in your mouth can mix into it thoroughly and have the necessary alkaline action upon it. This action turns insoluble starches into soluble sugars which can be absorbed by the body.

The tongue forms the food into a soft pulpy mass or bolus, to make it easier to swallow. When you bolt your food you can feel that large hard lump that has not been through this process of preparation. If your mother said to you, 'Don't bolt your food' when you were a child, this is why! The food is prevented from going up into the back of your nasal cavity by the soft palate, and from going down your windpipe into your lungs by a flap of tissue called the epiglottis. The epiglottis also controls the rate at which the food passes down your oesophagus into your stomach.

Food stays in your stomach for two or three hours while acidic gastric juices from the stomach walls break it down. Often people complain of having an 'acid tummy' and think, not always correctly, that they have eaten something that was too acidy or that had not 'agreed' with them. Many times this acid sensation in your stomach is caused by not having properly chewed your food. That first, alkaline action in your mouth was missed out or insufficient, so that when the food reached your stomach it received acid treatment that it had not, literally, been prepared for – and so you experience 'acid tummy' and general digestive discomfort.

From the stomach your food passes to your small intestine, into the first section called the duodenum. Here more secretions necessary for digestion come from the liver (via the gall bladder) and the pancreas. These juices are alkaline in action.

Your food is now fully treated and the nourishment it carries is ready for absorption into your blood stream.

Throughout the length of your alimentary tract, the rate of progress of food is controlled by the size and shape of the area it is passing through and by a series of muscles, some forming a flap or sphincter at the exit or entrance to the next passage or tube. This way your food is contained in any area long enough, during its preparation period, for digestive juices to act upon it; and during the absorption period for maximum nourishment to pass through the intestine walls into the blood tissues to be circulated throughout your body.

The ileum, or small intestine, lies coiled within your abdomen like one long piece of spaghetti. The mass of loops slows down and therefore controls the passage of your food, making the absorption period as long and complete as possible. At the junction of the ileum with your large intestine (the colon) is the ileo-caecal valve and if it stays 'closed' more than it should you will be aware of a 'pile-up' of matter in the lower right corner of your abdomen. Here often is the apparent starting point, although not necessarily the cause, of constipation. Once in the colon any remaining nourishment, mostly salts and water, passes through the walls and by the time it has reached the pelvic colon the contents are mostly solid. If the muscles and nerves that supply this area are not functioning correctly, this waste can often remain here longer than is healthy for you.

From the pelvic colon the solid matter, from which all nourishment has been taken, is stored in the rectum until it is expelled by the relaxation of the sphincter muscles of the anus.

Excretion, and temperature control

Every time you breathe out, you expel carbon dioxide and heat from your body. Other products of metabolism (see pages 74-5) that have to be removed are excess water, salts and substances produced by the breakdown of proteins, e.g. urea.

The kidneys excrete urea, salts and excess water as urine, which is passed to the bladder to be voided. The sweat glands of the skin also secrete salty water containing some urea. The evaporation of water from the skin is a continuous process and is not usually noticeable, unless you become hot, through exercise for example. The sweat glands then become more active, and as sweat evaporates it produces a cooling effect. Temperature regulation is in fact the chief function of the sweat glands.

Your skin regulates body temperature in yet another way. The tiny blood vessels near the skin surface dilate when you are hot, so the excess heat is rapidly got rid of through radiation. Conversely, if you are feeling cold, the skin vessels are constricted, and blood is diverted from the surface of the skin. The skin is then pale and cold, and sweating almost stops.

When you feel yourself getting chilly, your natural reaction is to get up and move around. The muscle action pumps blood faster and helps to warm you up. This is a deliberate action on your part, whereas when you shiver from cold the same thing happens but it is an involuntary action. Nature is also warning you that you are getting too cold and saying, 'Do something about it'.

Some people sweat more than others. The more you have exerted yourself the more noticeable the sweat will be. A lukewarm shower is a good way to refresh your skin and help you cool down. A really cold shower is too much of a shock to the system. It will make the tiny blood vessels in the skin close up, actually preventing heat loss.

If you tend only to sweat a little, you may find yourself going to the lavatory more frequently for a while after exercise, as this is yet another way of expelling waste products.

Good functioning of your kidneys is particularly important for waste elimination. The balance of heat, water and salts in your body must be maintained, and waste matter not lost in other ways becomes the overall responsibility of the kidneys (amongst their other functions, such as the regulation of blood pressure).

If your kidneys become strained at any time, you will be sensitive to this and find yourself placing your hands over them for comfort: on your back above your hips and just below your rib cage. Watch when you see other people doing this – you will notice they have their right hand a little lower than their left hand. This is because your right kidney lies lower in your body than your left kidney, leaving space to accommodate your liver which is almost directly above it.

Glands – *your passport to maturity*

The glandular system is fascinating and a vast study in itself, but a brief description is sufficient here.

There are two types of gland: exocrine and endocrine. Exocrine glands secrete through ducts onto a surface or cavity. Most glands are exocrine, e.g. sweat glands and digestive glands.

The endocrine or ductless glands secrete chemical messengers – hormones – in minute quantities directly from gland cells into the bloodstream. Hormones affect certain body parts or processes.

The chief endocrine glands are the pituitary gland, the thyroid and parathyroid glands, and the suprarenal or adrenal glands. Some body organs have an endocrine function as well as their other functions, e.g. stomach, pancreas, duodenum, kidneys, ovaries and testis.

The pituitary gland is at the base of your foreskull and for safe keeping is encased in its own bony cavity. It is the 'master' endocrine gland as the hormones it produces control many of the other endocrine glands.

The thyroid gland lies in your neck, just below your Adam's apple, and has two lobes. Its hormone, thyroxin, controls your general metabolism. Underactivity of the gland at birth causes cretinism in which mental and physical growth are retarded. In adults, deficiency of secretion causes sluggishness and puffy skin; excess produces nervousness and overactivity.

Behind each lobe of the thyroid gland are the two parathyroid glands. These help maintain the calcium levels in the blood.

The thymus gland lies behind your chest bone, or sternum. It is important in juvenile development, for growth and immunity.

There are two adrenal glands, one capping each kidney. The outer layer of the gland secretes steroid hormones which regulate your salt and water balance, affect metabolism and have an anti-inflammatory effect. The inner layer produces adrenaline at times of excitement or danger. Adrenaline is known as the 'get up and go' hormone because in situations of 'fright, flight or fight' your blood pressure rises and your muscles contract more readily to cope with the situation in which you find yourself.

The pancreas is a large gland adjacent to the duodenum. Besides producing digestive juice, it secretes the hormones insulin and glucagon which control the level of sugar in the blood.

The largest exocrine gland is the liver, which is situated in the uppermost part of the abdominal cavity on the right side beneath the diaphragm. Its functions are concerned with metabolism. It secretes bile (necessary for the digestion of fat).

Eastern thought puts forward the theory that the development, recession or dominance of the principle endocrine glands plays a vital role, possibly at seven-year intervals, in the development of certain aspects of your growing maturity and evolution as a human being. For example, the hormones from the thymus suppress the development of the sex organs until at puberty the recession of an active thymus allows the sex organs to develop, with the accompanying upheaval in a young person's physical, mental and emotional balance. About seven years later another gland becomes dominant in its function and purpose, bringing with it a maturing sense of responsibility to both yourself and life in general. At 21 years this used to be called 'coming of age' and an individual was thought responsible enough to cast a vote and marry without parental consent. This 'age' has been lowered to 18, but are we actually, at 18, sufficiently evolved or mature to cope with the responsibilities now put upon us?

By the age of 49 (7 x 7) in a normal, healthy person these seven endocrine glands have either served or are continuing to serve their purpose.You could be considered truly mature and wise; and if the experience of 49 years of living has been recognised and understood, you have much from the age of 50 to your demise to offer to your fellows and the world in general.

Jacques in Shakespeare's *As You Like It* says 'One man in his time plays many parts, His acts being seven ages . . . ' If you read on, remember though that the lifespan in Shakespeare's day was shorter than it is nowadays!

Nerves – *itch and you scratch*

Your nervous system is complex and without the intricate relaying of messages to and from your brain no other part of your body would work.

Your brain is the governing organ, the mastermind! It weighs about 1.5 kg/3 lb and is divided into several large sections, each having an overall responsibility for the functioning of specific areas of your body. For example, the cerebrum is the centre for memory, speech, vision, hearing etc.; the cerebellum coordinates voluntary muscle movement and balance; and the medulla oblongata, which forms the lower part of the brain stem, is the command centre for your breathing and circulation, both involuntary actions. The medulla oblongata is therefore vital to life. There, most of the descending motor nerve fibres from the brain cross from one side to the other. Thus the motor area of the right side of your brain controls the left side of your body and vice versa.

The spinal cord is continuous with the medulla oblongata; it is amply protected by the strong structure of your backbone. The individual bones, or vertebrae, of the spine are shaped and related to form a passage, the long, narrow spinal canal, through which the spinal cord passes, ending just where the lumbar vertebrae begin. The nerve fibres of the soinal cord emerge in bundles – the spinal nerves – through the gaps between the vetebrae.

There are 31 pairs of spinal nerves altogether, containing both sensory and motor nerve fibres. The spinal nerves divide again and again throughout the body, serving the various tissues. The head is served by 12 pairs of nerves (the 12 cranial nerves).

Nerve impulses from all parts of the body pass through your spinal cord which acts as a 'switchboard' for relaying messages to the brain for decision-making.

Sensory nerve fibres carry information about sensations, such as taste, irritation, cold, etc. Motor nerve fibres carry instructions away from the spinal cord to effect a suitable response.

Voluntary actions result from conscious activity by the brain. For example, if you get a speck of dust in your eye, sensory nerve fibres tell your brain what has happened. The brain instructs the motor nerves to activate the required muscles so that you can pull your hanky out of your pocket, walk to a mirror and remove the offending object.

In rapid, automatic reactions to sensory stimuli of an urgent nature, the neural pathway is 'short-circuited'. The messages pass to and from the spinal cord, by-passing the involvement of the brain. For example, you snatch your hand away if you touch something very hot, and you throw out your arms to keep your balance if someone pushes you. This is called reflex action.

Another type of involuntary nervous action is that controlling the inner organs, e.g. the digestive organs, cardio-vascular system, glands, and so on. This system is called the autonomic system and is subdivided into the sympathetic system and the parasympathetic system. Many organs receive nerve fibres from both systems which may act antagonistically. For example, peristalsis (waves of contraction) is stimulated in the muscles of the gut by the parasympathetic supply and is inhibited by the sympathetic supply.

If damage or injury occurs to any of the spinal or cranial nerves, there will be lack of sensation and/or power at the parts of the body they serve.

One seemingly remote reaction is when injury occurs to the nerves at the base of your neck. Nerves radiating out as high as this serve the large pair of back muscles called latissimus dorsi. Latissimus dorsi (one muscle each side of your spine) originates as low down your back as the crest of your hip bone. It inserts into a groove in the bone in the top of each arm. One of its actions is to help you to lift your lower body by using your arms, for example when walking with crutches or climbing. Damage and malfunction at neck level to the motor nerves supplying this large muscle could prevent you from doing these actions and could result in paralysis at this lower part of your body.

One of the pieces of equipment in a multi-gym is called 'the latissimus station' because, when you use it, it is the latissimus dorsi muscle you are exercising. If you watch someone at latissimus station you will clearly see the belly of this muscle bulging as it works.

The balancing act

Obviously no one body system can exist without interrelating with all the others. In a healthy person, especially a young child with few pressures and demands, each system is in balance with itself and also with the others to create a whole, healthy human being. Unfortunately as you get older the demands made upon you, your reactions to them, and any irregularities that may result from this, can disturb the balance.

Nature is always balancing and rebalancing for you and it is very important to understand and remember this. Too often in a desire to heal or mend, you dose yourself up in one way or another; if you left things alone nature would do it for you. You may be making her job harder, and the result for many people can be that their natural immune system becomes less effective in time of real need. Instead of being resistant to a virus or infection, you can – by over-use of antibiotics, for example – weaken your natural immune system so much that you succumb to an infection when you might not otherwise have done so.

The same principle of altering nature's balance applies with the zealous taking of extra vitamins, especially in the winter. If you are healthy and follow a sound, balanced diet, you don't require these supplements and by taking them you are doing yourself a disservice; a balanced diet should provide all the vitamins and minerals you require. You would also do well to remember that most Western people tend too eat too much. Even when all the nutritional requirements are catered for in a balanced diet, if you eat more than your body needs you are putting a further demand on your system, to balance, to eliminate, or to store as excess fat. You only need to eat enough to maintain your health and to provide the energy required for the lifestyle you have chosen.

For more about nutrition, turn to the next section.

Chapter 3

Feeding the system: NUTRITION

*T*hat the digestive system should work well is more important than you probably realise, and it's possibly the system of the body that you treat with least respect.

Why you eat

You eat for three reasons: to build up your body, to make good wear and tear, and to provide fuel for the production of heat and energy. If your digestive system isn't working properly these three functions won't be satisfactory. A chain reaction may set in: your body doesn't grow as intended, nor replenish or mend itself; your body temperature doesn't regulate as and when it should; and you become not only generally tired but lack the energy to get through the day's activities effectively. This in turn leads to general malaise, susceptibility to illness or disease, irritation and bad temper, poor concentration and circulation; which in turn could be responsible for lower mental and physical performance, accidents, periods of ill health, impatience and inability to consider or understand other people, arguments, general inability to cope, early old age.

So it is essential to ensure that your digestive system works properly. Which means, more than anything else, that you've got to put into it the nutrition that will help it: quality food and a properly balanced diet (which does not necessarily mean, thank goodness, expensive eating habits).

Nutrition, its content and value and your individual requirements, is a vast and complex subject. So much literature is available that you may not know where to start! It's also too easy to get so involved with working out what you should or should not eat, for whatever reason, that it just becomes too complicated to bother, or the whole thing gets out of proportion and you become obsessive and fanatical about it – and boring!

So I have set out, as simply as possible, your average nutritional requirements and the foods in which these requirements can be found, followed by a simple golden rule for you to follow.

The character of food

Your nutritional requirements

Protein is essential for growth, repair and reproduction. It is the only class of food containing nitrogen. If you cut down too drastically on protein you will experience a negative nitrogen balance, and will lose not only the fat content of your muscles but the required lean tissue, i.e. strong muscles which you need to move around and for all physical activities.

Protein is found in animal products: meat, fish, eggs, milk and cheese (class A proteins); and cereals, pulses and gelatin (class B proteins).

Carbohydrates are essential for creating heat and energy. They are mostly eaten as starches and sugars.

Starches are produced by green plants, stored in the

stems, roots and seeds, and are available as cereals, nuts, root vegetables and the stems and stalks of green vegetables. (The outer leaves of green vegetables are often the most nutritious and tasty, but, because they are usually trimmed away by the retailers, we can often only buy 'tidy' vegetables. Never discard more than you need of vegetables when you prepare them.)

Sugars are found in cane, beet, honey and fruit. There are many types of sugar. Refined sugar has no nutritional value other than the calories, or energy potential, it provides.

Starches undergo a chemical change during digestion, turning into types of sugar which the body can absorb.

Fats are used to produce heat and energy. They are the chief reservoir of energy, also storing the vital fat-soluble vitamins A, D, E and K. They help to hold your body organs and nerve tissues in place and to protect them from injury. They help to prevent skin rashes and to promote healing. They insulate your body for essential warmth. With a list like that, you can see that sufficient fat intake is vital. In Western countries, however, our intake of fat is generally too high, and we would benefit from a reduced fat intake, especially of saturated fats which are found particularly in meat and dairy products.

Vegetable fats mainly are found in some fruits (e.g. olive, avocado) and a variety of seeds and nuts (e.g. sunflower, walnut). Most are rich in unsaturated fats, though coconut and palm oil contain a high proportion of saturated fats.

Water forms two-thirds of your body weight. It is essential to life itself, and lack of water is more immediately serious than lack of food. Water is present in every cell and involved in every process in your body, from the most obvious, such as your liquid blood, to the very structure of your bodily cells. Your water balance must be maintained so that the amount gained is equal to the amount lost. Your body controls this for you: any excess not used by the body is passed in the urine.

In addition to the water we drink, water is found in fruit and vegetables; for example potatoes are 75 per cent water.

Minerals are an essential part of your diet, but are required in minute quantities so a sound diet which balances the major food components is usually sufficient in minerals. Some of the major ones include the following.

Calcium is essential for growth, strong bones and teeth and blood clotting. It is found in milk, cheese, egg yolk and vegetables, especially carrots and cabbage.

Iodine balances your metabolic processes and is essential to your thyroid gland. It is found in seafood.

Iron is essential for the production of red blood cells. It is found in red meat, eggs, cheese, bread and green vegetables.

Magnesium ensures the healthy function of the heart, the arterial system and the kidneys, and is needed for bone formation and the control of pre-menstrual tension. It is found in bread, grain products, cocoa, seafood and pulses.

Phosphorus is required for the production of muscular and nervous energy and for the correct composition of your bones and teeth. It is found in milk, egg yolks and green vegetables.

Sodium chloride and potassium regulate the fluid balance in the body and are found in most foods.

Sulphur is needed for the well-being of all your tissues and is found in all proteins.

Vitamins are essential to life, health, growth and proper metabolism. There are 13 major vitamins. Vitamins A, D, E and K are fat soluble and can be stored in the body. Vitamin C and the eight vitamins that make up the B complex are water soluble and should be taken daily. (Vitamin B_{12} can be stored in the liver.) Vitamins work together with mineral salts: for example, iron can only be absorbed if vitamin C is present in the body. Fortunately, a balanced diet should ensure an adequate daily vitamin intake, except at special times during childhood, pregnancy and old age when you may need a boost of certain vitamins. Your doctor or child care clinic will tell you which ones. Avoid dosing yourself up with unnecessary vitamin supplements, which are expensive and may in rare cases be harmful if you are prescribing for yourself.

Fibre is essential in your diet because it absorbs and retains water, forming a bulk to assist the passage of food through the digestive tract. If you have a tendency to diarrhoea or constipation you will find fibrous food a great help. But there's no need to go over the top, including an excessive amount of fibre, or you'll begin to put on weight! Excess fibre also inhibits vitamin and mineral uptake and may *cause* constipation. You only need enough!

Many foods that you eat daily are fibrous in character: unrefined grains, peas and beans, potatoes, uncooked fruit and vegetables (including lettuce).

Additives

If you eat a balanced diet with food as fresh as possible, non-refined, not pre-frozen, raw where you like it and, when cooked, preferably eaten the same day, additives should not be necessary. This includes salt because salt occurs naturally in most foods you eat. If you add salt 'to bring out the flavour' then you are probably eating food that has lost its freshness and some of its goodness and you are trying to recapture flavour for your palate. Heavy smoking, drinking and meat-eating can ruin your palate's ability to detect flavours.

Food when frozen or cooked undergoes chemical changes, altering its nutritional content. If you cook it for too long or in too much water, a large percentage of the goodness will pass from the food into the water which you then throw down the sink! If you peel your vegetables (especially potatoes) and many fruits you are again throwing away nutritional value. It's not going to do your drains or dustbin any good, but could have made a lot of difference to you!

Food that has been prepared and treated for sale in shops usually contains at least some additives. This can be checked by looking at the label on the tin or package. A healthy body does not need these additives, but can easily cope with a limited quantity.

If you think your diet contains too many unnecessary additives you need to change your habit of shopping, preparing and eating your food for your diet to become wholesome and balanced. There is an enormous selection available to suit your individual palate and fancy. Change can be a real challenge and fun! But it is not easy for everyone. If you find it difficult, go about things gradually. Start by changing to wholemeal bread and cutting out shop-prepared meals, then make small changes each week to improve your diet in stages.

Mix and match

There are types of food which do not mix together. When you eat them at the same meal they set up incompatible chemical reactions in your stomach. These foods are not otherwise 'bad' for you, but your digestive system has to overcome and sort out an intake which does not match. If you experience discomfort after certain meals, check what you have eaten against the following golden rule, based on the Hay system pioneered at the beginning of the century by Dr William Hay.

Do not mix together, at the same meal, proteins and acid fruit with starches and sugars.

When to eat

Three meals a day is generally accepted as being what the human system requires, but there are no hard and fast rules because we are all individual. There is no reason why you should eat breakfast soon after you get up and before you go to work, if you are not hungry. Unfortunately at the time of the morning when you may need to break your fast you may be in a job situation that prevents you from doing this. The real rule is to eat when you are hungry and to stop eating when you are no longer hungry. (Likewise to drink only when you are thirsty.) If you keep strictly to that rule you will probably be healthy and find you are eating much less. Nibbling between meals is not a sin but it keeps your digestive system working all the time, and that too needs a rest. The energy required from you to work your digestive system is considerable and could be put towards other functions, for example the important function of healing should you be under the weather or ill. The healing process will be more effective and quicker if your energy can be concentrated towards that one function. You won't starve or suffer if you stop eating for longer periods than you are accustomed.

Don't, however, eat your last major meal late at night, or if you do, leave a good space of time before you go to bed. Your digestive system has come to the end of the day too! Although it goes on working for you at all times it also needs a rest and after a day's work it too finds the going harder and its efforts may also keep you from sleeping. It's not the cheese that keeps you awake but the fact that cheese takes a lot of digesting. It's sleep-time, not digesting-time. Most proteins and dairy produce require a lot of digesting in order to get full nutritional benefit from them, so eat them earlier in the day to put their benefits to use during the day when your body needs them most.

Balance and individuality

The important theme throughout every section of this book is balance and individuality. Where food is concerned, firstly eat when your system indicates and what you like. Try not to put together incompatible foods. Eat in moderation. Eat each class of food in moderation (too much meat protein can give you acidity, too much raw vegetable can give you flatulence). A balanced diet is considered to be one that contains essential nutrients in suitable proportions. Ideally, your daily intake should balance out at about 11 per cent protein, 30 per cent fat (no more than one-third of which should be hard unsaturated fat) and 59 per cent carbohydrate (grain or vegetable products).

Remember that individual requirements differ: one man's meat is another man's poison. If your child says he cannot finish his meal or does not like what is on his plate, he may not be being difficult, his system may not be able to cope with the food or the quantity. A child will instinctively stop eating something 'wrong' much quicker than an adult. We often ignore our bodies and carry on eating through habit, good manners or greed! Respect what your child is trying to tell you because he probably doesn't know how to explain his problem, and as he gets older he may simply not want to be told off at 'leaving his food'.

Individual requirements are also affected by your environment, age, sex, size, the climate, your clothing and the nature of your work. If your metabolic rate is slow you will probably require less food and if it is quick you may require a greater intake at each meal, or meals more frequently, or both.

Unless you have something medically wrong with you (in which case you should be receiving appropriate treatment) or you know that your diet is very unbalanced, that you eat immoderately, or are very overweight or underweight there is no need to go into your dietary requirements in depth. All you need to understand is that your system requires a balance of all the major food types in sensible quantities, and also that you should enjoy your food. If you eat to live you will find the right balance, but if you live to eat then you are creating a big problem for yourself.

Not all that long ago, nutritional knowledge that is now commonplace had not even been 'discovered' by our scientists and nutritionists. Yet men and women who ate a balanced, moderate diet were just as healthy in their ignorance as we are today with all the mind-boggling information available to us. We can be 'blinded by science' – facts, lists, charts, graphs in every book you pick up about food, especially where 'slimming' is concerned. It is quite possible that our food contains many more nutritional qualities than we are yet aware of, so opinions about what we should eat may change again and again. But if you are eating a balanced, moderate diet containing plenty of fresh foods which keeps you happy, healthy and fit, why not just carry on as you are? It all boils down to the proof of the pudding!

Chapter 4

A new shape:
SLIMMING

*W*eight fluctuates from day to day and from morning to evening due to the rate of your metabolism, whether or not you are menstruating, and even the time of year. Most of us must expect to see a difference of 1-1½ kg/2-3 lb over a week. However, if we are honest we also know when we are overweight.

Face the facts

It is a hard fact that if you eat less and if you eat the right foods, you will weigh less: but eating less is easier said than done, and before you embark on any slimming regime, you must take a good hard look at your personality, your reasons for being overweight, why you want to lose weight, and what will be the most successful way for you, personally, to achieve weight loss.

What is your aim?

According to your present size and weight, be realistic. Do you want to shed a little or do you need to lose a lot?

Have a target in mind that you can achieve. If you are tall and big-boned, you'll never look like a Barbie doll! It's also important to be happy. If you are striving for something completely out of your reach, you'll only feel frustrated and disappointed.

Your ideal weight does not have to relate to your age and height. Most of all it should relate to your state of mind and temperament. The weight, size and shape at which you know you feel good, function well and feel happy is what to aim for and maintain. So think about what you need to do. Do you want to shape yourself but otherwise stay the same weight? Do you only want to tone up slack muscles? Do you want to lose weight to get into your clothes again? Or all of these?

The limits of success

You must realise that your achievements are limited by bone structure and metabolism.

Your basic bone structure is genetic and cannot be altered. To find your frame size measure around your wrist: 13 cm/5½ in is a small frame; 13-17 cm/5½-6½ in is a medium frame; 17 cm/6½ in and over is a large frame. A larger frame is more likely to be overweight and there's a limit to how much you can lose. You have to start by accepting your frame size and your basic bone structure.

Your natural rate of metabolism affects your slimming success, but is not absolutely fixed. It is influenced by your eating and exercising habits, your body size, age, sex, the climate, environment, the type of clothes you wear and the nature of your work. Nervous tension affects your breathing and heart rate and thus your rate of metabolism.

If you have a slow metabolic rate, your food is converted less into energy and heat and more into fat. The right exercise will speed up a slow metabolic rate, in which case you may start to lose some weight regardless of your food intake, providing you are already eating sensibly. A quick metabolic rate means that your food is converted more into energy and heat and less into fat, so you are less likely to be prone to overweight.

Your success rate will be slower if you are overtired, tense or seriously in need of a break or a holiday. These should be sorted out first. It is not wise to embark on a slimming regimen when feeling like this. You will only make yourself feel worse and almost certainly fail in your objectives.

If you are considerably overweight or oversize, success will of course take longer than if you have only a little to lose.

Why are you overweight?

Be honest. Is it one of these?

One of the most common causes of people being overweight is wrong eating habits. Change them! You may not be eating food that satisfies you or gives your body its required nutritional needs because you are too calorie conscious, not interested in food, or being lazy.

Another common problem is simply eating too much. If you enjoy food to excess, you must learn to eat moderately! Eat to live rather than live to eat. If you continue over-eating, you will get fatter, heavier, more shapeless, ungainly, less able to move around and become susceptible to heart and respiratory problems.

Fluid retention is not unusual, giving a bloated feeling sometimes accompanied by flatulence and burping. This produces extra inches rather than extra weight but is distressing. It's often caused or aggravated by a slow metabolic rate and can be more difficult to overcome than other causes. If you are seriously affected, you should discuss it with your doctor. Otherwise, keep off chocolates, cakes, sweets and processed foods and reduce your salt intake to a minimum. A short, controlled fast or semi-fast may help to sort out the problem. Exercise is essential: all-over exercise, especially curling and stretching and the warm-up sequence couldn't be better for you.

Comfort eating is very common. It not only produces overweight, it can produce feelings of guilt which make you eat more – a vicious circle which can be hard to escape. But the first step is to do away with those feelings of guilt. Comfort eating can be caused by the most human of reasons: being tired, depressed, bored, lonely, tense, lacking confidence, being unoccupied, self-pity. Think hard about the cause in your case and take steps to sort it out; you must, and not just for your shape or weight problem. Take a long look at yourself and your lifestyle: a change could be as good as a diet. If you are bored, join a club, an exercise class or take up a hobby. If you are lacking in confidence, decide what you do best and try to learn more about that area or improve your skills to give yourself more self-esteem. Look at the many opportunities available and take them. It can be hard, but only you can take the appropriate action to get off the merry-go-round. Once you do, food will become less important. Understanding why you comfort eat is an enormous step towards successfully stopping it.

Taking control

The most effective way of changing your eating habits is to cleanse your system and your palate. Break the eating pattern and your attitude to it and in so doing you can alter that pattern for the better. Make a decision on when you will eat, what foods you will choose and how you will prepare them. Treat yourself to a new and appropriate cookery book and plan your meals rather than deciding in a haphazard fashion what the next meal will be.

You have to be in control. This can be hard for some people, but don't belittle yourself. You can do it. If you take pride in the fact that you control your own self, your desires and your body, it's more than the first step to success.

Don't make resolutions. Be honest. If you force a diet you will become frustrated, tense, perhaps break it, binge, feel guilty, and then you have to start all over again! Leave it until a more appropriate time or try a less rigorous approach.

You are not helped by all the advertising – ignore it! Nor by the abundance of chocolates, sweets, cakes and biscuits strategically placed in shops and newsagents. Recognise this; they are after all trading on your weakness, that's why they do it! Write a shopping list before you go out and stick to it rigidly. Above all, never shop when you are hungry.

Once you have achieved your new eating pattern, listen to your system, and eat as it dictates and not as your brain remembers. Keep your intake light, small and balanced. Don't let yourself slip back into old habits or ways of thinking or feeling. Changing eating habits requires determination, self-discipline, will-power, pride and pleasure in who you are and what you are doing. You can achieve it!

Your kind of slimming diet

There are so many slimming diets around, it is often hard to choose between them. They all seem to claim success, but you should remember that the success is related only to you and your eating habits, not to the diet itself. It is therefore important to choose a way of eating which suits your way of life, your level of will-power and your schedule. Think about your patterns of eating and your expectations and consider what sort of diet would be most suitable.

Would you benefit from a crash diet to give you encouragement, or are you better aiming for a slower weight loss?

Do you like to eat early or late? If early, are you tempted to go on eating? If late, how late? You must have time and some gentle exercise between your last meal and going to bed. Do you feel out of sorts when you wake up, or about one hour after getting up? This indicates that you are eating too late and too close to bedtime. Can you change your mealtimes or bedtime? The change may do a lot of good.

When you start eating, do you find it difficult to stop? Discipline is required. Use some of the psychological 'gimmicks' on pages 59-62 to help you. They work!

Do you keep a calorie count? If you do, do you become a calorie bore, always thinking and talking about calorie values of foods and perhaps neglecting their quality?

Do you like to change your menu regularly or stick to the same one while you are dieting?

Find a slimming diet which suits you best, but remember that the best way to diet is to change to new, sensible eating habits, eat good food and eat less.

When to diet

When you are relaxed is the best time to diet.

You should diet at a time when you are most likely to succeed. It can be at any time of the year when you have a strong incentive. Lent is often a favourable time as this 'external' control can help back up your will power. Before Christmas is also a good time, rather than afterwards!

When a 'bandwagon' comes along – jump on it. The 'bandwagon' is possibly an instinct, a natural directive from your body – answer it. Everything will fall into place and become easier. If you don't answer it, you cannot tell when or if it will occur again.

When not to diet

Don't embark on a slimming diet if your body has other, more important things to do. Don't diet if you are pregnant, if you are ill or tired. If you have a medical condition or are taking medication, for diabetes or cancer, for example, discuss your plans and intentions with your doctor. Don't give blood during a slimming diet.

What to expect when you diet

When dieting, your body is readjusting, that is all. You may experience reactions to this adjustment, but there should be no cause for alarm. These reactions are only temporary but must occur, when you consider what is happening. Your system is cleansing and rebalancing; tensions and bad habits that have formed, whether physical or mental, have to make way for something different. The reactions are positive signs that change is occurring, so be encouraged.

Reactions you may experience:

- dizziness, headaches, feeling of faintness
- fatigues, weakness
- shivery, cold
- nausea
- bad breath, coated tongue.

When dieting avoid hot baths, sustained exercise (such as jogging, running, trampolining) sudden movements (jumping up suddenly). These could aggravate any of the reactions from the above list. If you are not sure, consult your GP.

If your stomach grumbles you may not really be in need of food, but your brain pattern is used to sending out 'feed me' signals at certain times of the day. You will soon recognise the difference between your brain pattern habits and real need. When the need for nutrition is real, your system as opposed to your brain memory is asking for nutrition (and not fish and chips or sweets!).

Your brain memory

From the earliest moments of your life your brain remembers. It remembers the pathways through your nervous system that pain takes. It remembers the pattern of feeding when you were an infant. For example, a baby that is breast-fed will stop suckling when he has had enough, but when he is bottle-fed or being weaned there is a temptation on the part of the parent to shovel that little bit that's left in the bottle or on the spoon down baby (even though he has indicated that he's had enough) and then say 'There's a good baby, to finish up all your food'! We often take away his self-control and hey presto! at this tender age bad habits have started. As an adult your brain remembers that you feed at certain times and that your palate likes certain foods. You often don't need many of the foods that you eat and you rarely need as much, but you listen to your brain memory rather than tuning in to your system's requirements.

You have to break this brain memory pattern and then re-educate yourself to a new way of thinking and doing in order to succeed.

Help yourself!

Dieting is always easier said than done, but here are some practical approaches that work. You have to be determined to succeed. Get rid of your scales and tape measure. Use your clothes and your silhouette in the mirror, as a guide to your improving shape.

Keep busy: make a list of all those jobs that have piled up and work through them all.

Remember – positive thinking! Not, I wish I were thin but, it will be nice when . . . Say, I can do it! regularly, or better still, *I am doing it!*

Find an absorbing interest so that you forget to eat – then you'll eat only when you're hungry and not in between meals. Return to work straight after eating.

Avoid introspection. Find interests outside yourself.

Do the warm-up sequence as soon as possible after waking. If you are feeling sluggish, it's a temptation to eat. The warm-up sequence will shake up your metabolism and get you going, your outlook and attitude will change and your resolve will strengthen.

You don't have to eat at socially conventional times: breakfast, lunch and supper. If friends say: have a drink or something to eat, say to yourself: Do I need it? If not, say no. If they press you against your will, the ill-manners are theirs, not yours. The same applies if you are dining out and are offered second helpings.

Eat only when you are hungry, that is, don't eat if you are not hungry. Recognise the difference between real hunger and mental gnawing pains. It's a different sensation.

Stop eating as soon as the hunger is satisfied and not when you feel full or have emptied your plate.

Wash up immediately, forget it, get on with something else.

Change your approach: aim to eat as little as possible to stay fit and healthy. After all, it's all your body needs!

Use a smaller plate. Present your food attractively and serve less. Sit down, relax and enjoy your meal.

Eat slowly and chew well (that's what your teeth are for!). You will find that you eat less. Well-chewed food is digested better, you need less and feel better. This is a fact.

Don't drink with your food.

Don't cook more than you need. (Don't give any leftovers to the dog or he will get fat!)

Try not to have in the house the things that you are avoiding.

If you are likely to forget what you've had during the day, write it down as you go along.

Don't think of yourself as dieting but as eating only when you need. Say, Do I *need* this? The only good reason for eating is if you are hungry.

Make your own routine and stick to it: eat at set times, say 8 a.m., 1 p.m., 6 p.m. Don't drink after, say, 8 p.m. You'll be up in the night; broken sleep leads to tiredness next day and you'll then eat more because you're tired or out of sorts.

Don't let yourself become tired or cold, or you will eat to regain the energy and heat that your body needs.

Don't eat between meals, it's a mental and physical reminder of food.

If you think you want to eat, sip water instead. It can do the trick.

If you absolutely have to nibble at something between meals, try a piece of celery or a carrot and chew them. Chewing takes time.

If you can't cope with celery or carrots, chew gum. If you choose a sugar-free gum it also cleans your teeth. You can make a piece of gum last a long time, but remember that other people may find it unsociable if you are talking and chewing at the same time.

If you feel you need something sweet, eat white grapes. Their calorie value is low, they are a natural aid to slimming and they will satisfy your longing for sweetness. Too many may give you tummy-ache!

You can *not* eat limitless amounts of fresh or raw fruit, vegetables and salad. Not only will the calories mount up, albeit slowly, but too much will produce acidity, flatulence or indigestion. Your diet will also no longer be balanced.

Decide whether you will talk about your slimming efforts or keep totally silent and let the results show for you – one approach or the other is right for you.

Never go shopping when you are hungry. You may find yourself having that quick mid-morning snack in a coffee bar, because you feel 'empty', or *think* you do.

Avoid all convenience foods.

Don't add salt to your food.

Grill, don't fry.

Use low-calorie fats on your bread, and 'butter' only one half of sandwiches.

Replace full fat milk with skimmed milk or semi-skimmed milk. And of course skimmed milk comes in powdered form too.

Replace marmalade and jams with low calorie diabetic marmalades and jams, or marmite and cottage cheese.

Don't lick the bowl after cooking!

Avoid constipation at all times and especially during a diet. Always clear constipation before you start a diet.

Don't eat late at night. If you think you will not sleep unless you have that little something just before bed, well, this is psychological isn't it? Be firm with yourself and abstaining will soon become a good habit. Let your body readjust naturally.

Keep a clean palate. If you get rid of the taste after each time you eat or drink you fool your brain memory! Clean your teeth and tongue after every intake. Don't use toothpaste – it has its own flavour. Just use water.

Finally, if you think you want to eat, instead lie down and relax for a few minutes. A mentally relaxed person requires less food.

How to slim safely and effectively

If your dog sits around all day and eats everything he can get, he will get fat – so would you. If you decide to slim him down, you do it by giving him regular, fairly demanding exercise (perhaps gently introduced) and less but balanced feeding with no snacks. He gets thinner, tones and shapes – so would you. His food and exercise are controlled by you – *so is yours!* The difference, of course, is that he has no option. But the results occur because they have to. So once you have resolved to lose weight and have the necessary determination, you will need self-control and will-power.

The following diets are all balanced. They follow your body's natural system and its healthy nutritional requirements. This makes them safe. They are neither a new approach nor a current fad, but are based on sound ideas and common sense. Remember you are only trying to lose excess fatty tissue, not lean tissue, so you must follow a balanced regime that respects your body and the way you use it. The following methods will all be effective and safe if you undertake them correctly. The only question is which one suits you best.

Once you have decided on your diet, organise yourself, think as little as you can about it and just get on with it. In other words, it should take up as small a part of your day as possible – everything else is more important.

When your initial slimming diet is finished, it will be easier to continue the good work as your eating habits will already have improved.

1. Eat less

This is a long-term successful diet. Ensure that your present diet is well balanced. If it is not, you will need to change your menus. Then, simply cut down on your intake: eat less of everything. This is a more family-orientated diet because you can all eat the same food, it's only you who cuts down the quantity.

For example, here are some methods of approach for you to consider:

If you usually eat three potatoes, take two. If two, take one – and so on with everything. Or you can eat a proportion, say half or two-thirds, of everything, including the number of cups of tea or coffee per day.

Ration out your food: one apple per day, half in the morning, half later on. Drink half a cup of tea or coffee at a time.

Use dessertspoons where you used to use tablespoons; use teaspoons where you used to use dessertspoons.

Eat only one of everything: one potato, one tomato, one slice of bread, one apple, one helping of vegetables etc., each day.

Since you can't halve your plate, use a smaller one!

2. Fast and break-fast

Overnight when you are asleep you are abstaining from food for the longest period in each 24 hours. During that time you are resting your system so that sleep, healing and the general cleansing and refreshing of your system is most effective. After waking, the first meal of the day, breakfast, is just that.

If you undertake a short fast all you are doing is extending the overnight abstinence from food in order to increase all these benefits. You limit your intake to water, which is essential.

Fasting is *not* starving. It is drinking only water and eating nothing for a *limited* period of time. This gives your system a rest and is the quickest way to break unwanted habits of eating. It also is the best way of discovering why you have been eating as you have and which foods or drinks have caused any ailments like headaches, migraine, sinus congestion, indigestion, kidney discomfort and so on. Fasting cleans out *all* systems, especially your alimentary system. Because a certain amount of sodium is removed from your body during a fast, your fatty tissues shrink and then tone up. When you reintroduce solid food, you are re-educating your brain pattern and letting your system dictate your eating habits.

For each day that you fast you must take one day to reintroduce food, as described later. A three-day fast is therefore a six-day controlled period. If you are an 'all-or-nothing' person you may find one, two or three days of fasting easy but have difficulty with the next three days of reintroduction. After this it takes a lot of self-control not to binge. If you think you may be like this, try the 'semi-fast' which requires no reintroduction days and can be continued for longer.

Who should not fast?

Some people should not fast. If in doubt, talk with your doctor about your weight, size or condition. You must not fast:

● if you are pregnant or have just had your baby. Also, if you are trying to become pregnant;

● if you have a medical condition;

● if you are taking any prescribed medication.

If you are very thin, or elderly, a *short* fast may be possible but not without the permission and supervision of your doctor.

How to fast

If necessary start your fast with a laxative the previous night, to give yourself a headstart.

Drink water only. Eat nothing. Water flushes out toxins and waste matter. It maintains the fluid balance in your body. It relieves, initially, any 'hunger pangs' that your brain may experience until such time as these 'hunger pangs' cease.

Drink about eight glasses of tepid water daily. As your body reacts, some of this water may be eliminated as urine, excessive to your previous quantity lost daily; or, imperceptibly, through the pores of your skin, thus keeping your fluid balance correct for you. Mineral or tap water are best.

Gentle exercise is excellent during your fast but do not participate in any form of sustained exercising such as jogging. Avoid sudden movements (like getting quickly out of bed or up from a chair) and don't take hot baths. Your blood pressure alters during a fast and you may experience a little dizziness. Moderation is the name of the game. There is no reason why your daily routine should otherwise alter in any way.

Reactions to your fast

Although the majority of people fast without discomfort of any kind, at the beginning you *may* experience what appear to be side-effects but which are really healthy signs that your fast is becoming effective. These reactions may be the occasional headache, dizziness, nausea, faintness or sense of chill. Your system is clearing itself of waste. If you are anxious about any of these reactions, talk with your doctor.

To begin with you may experience a 'gnawing' feeling in your stomach but this is simply your digestive system readjusting itself. Sip a little water. Your tongue may become coated and your breath may smell a little but again these are signs of your system eliminating and readjusting to better overall health. They are good signs of success. You can keep your mouth and breath fresh by cleaning your teeth, scraping your tongue and gargling, but with *water*. Don't use anything flavoured. These 'symptoms' will recede and when your tongue and breath are pleasant again nature is telling you that the time has come to break your fast. Do not take vitamin tablets while fasting as they will activate the digestive system.

How to break your fast and introduce new eating patterns

On the first day, dilute four glasses of orange or apricot juice with your eight glasses of water, i.e. one part of juice to two parts of water. Sip small but frequent amounts throughout the entire day, making it last until evening. (Do not substitute apple juice as it is too acid.)

On the second day (if you have fasted for two days), drink four glasses of undiluted juice and four glasses of water throughout the day, at two-hour intervals.

On the third day (if you have fasted for three days), continue with the same liquid intake. Include a little grated apple in plain yoghurt, eating small amounts of this every three hours.

On subsequent days, continue with the same liquid intake. Introduce solid food in very small and digestible quantities, carefully increasing the amount each day, still three-hourly. Choose from: grated apple, grated carrot, plain yoghurt, honey, crispbread, cereal, wholemeal bread, cottage cheese, potatoes. This slowly reintroduces a balanced diet of fats, carbohydrates and proteins.

Don't go back to your old eating habits or you might as well not have bothered!

An excellent book has been written about fasting. It is called *Fasting: The Ultimate Diet* and is by Dr Allan Cott, with Jerome Agel and Eugene Boe. It goes into the business of fasting in great detail with many fascinating explanations. Unfortunately it is currently out of print, so keep an eye open for it in your local library, second-hand bookshops or at jumble sales.

Once you have reached your goal, maintain it with a regular 24-hour fast each week, on the same day of the week. This period of fasting includes your night time sleep. After the evening meal before your chosen day of the week, drink water only, no food until your evening meal the next day. This is complete 24-hour rest from food and drink (other than water). It maintains your weight, rests your digestive system, cleanses your system and includes your all-healing sleep period. On the other six days of the week – eat sensibly!

3. Semi-fast

This isn't true fasting, because during a semi-fast you are eating solids and drinking liquids other than water only. The principle is only to drink during the day and then to eat a very light, small meal early in the evening, which must be nutritious and, of course, balanced.

On the first day, during the day, take warmed water

only, about six glasses. Decide on a time for your evening meal, say 6 p.m. or 7 p.m. and stick to that time each day. Keep this evening meal light, small and easily digestible – something like cottage cheese, scrambled egg, plain yoghurt with an accompaniment of salad or vegetables. Enjoy a cup of coffee or tea afterwards if that is what you like. Drink no more after about 8 p.m. to ensure unbroken sleep. You need good quality sleep during any diet programme.

Subsequent days should follow a similar pattern. However you vary your menu, keep to the rule of light, small, easily digestible meals.

If at any time you find yourself in need of extra energy during the day, an orange (full of vitamin C) will give you a quick release of energy and an apple (full of vitamin E) will give you a slow release of energy. Or drink pure fruit juice instead.

As with true fasting, continue with your usual exercising pattern providing that you do not undertake any sustained exercise such as jogging, aerobics or working in the gym. This is where walking comes into its own. Again, avoid sudden movements and hot baths because your blood pressure alters and you may experience a little dizziness.

There is no reintroduction period for a semi-fast; you can gradually reintroduce, say, three meals a day if that is how you prefer to eat, providing you keep to the principles of better eating habits. Again, results may be dramatic initially and steady down as the days pass. There should be no need to consult your doctor if you keep to the principles of the diet as long as you do not have any of the following contra-indications. Do not diet if:

● you are pregnant or have just had your baby. Also, if you are trying to become pregnant;

● if you have a medical condition;

● if you are taking any prescribed medication.

4. Weight Watchers

Weight Watchers is a well-established organisation with well-proven case histories and results. They usually advertise in your local newspaper and you pay for the instruction. The dieting is supervised with care, individual attention and encouragement and the methods of dieting are balanced and gentle to your system. Weight Watchers is very suitable if you are very overweight and have been for a long time.

5. Don't mix foods that fight

This is the Hay system, a way of eating that has produced good health for many people. They have experienced permanent better health and increased energy, and many have lost unwanted weight in the process. The principle is at each meal only to eat foods that are compatible with each other. Dr Hay's method is described in *Food Combining for Health* and the majority of recipes in the book are vegetarian, a preference of eating that is given little or no space in most books on weight loss or shape control.

Energy input *versus* energy output

This book does not include a calorie-countdown because its approach to shaping, slimming and toning incorporates an overall lifestyle of exercising, eating, knowledge of your body structure and function and an understanding of your personality and temperament. If, however, you feel you need a calorie count there are endless sources of information available. But remember, if you keep a calorie count you will be thinking about it, talking about it, and have it endlessly on your mind.

If you are not in a position to undertake other forms of exercise you should be able to do the warm-up sequence and to walk. Because walking is available to nearly everyone, it is taken here as the best example of the ratio of exercise with the burning up of energy calories.

When you walk briskly for one minute you burn up approximately five calories. One hour 40 minutes of brisk walking per week burns up 500 calories per week. Per year this will keep off 3 kg/8 lb! This is providing that you are not putting in more than you are burning up (i.e. more food than your body *needs*) or you will of course alter the balance.

The following guide indicates approximately how many calories you burn up, per minute, with other forms of exercise, compared with sitting still.

Activity	Calories per minute
Walking upstairs	20
Running	14
Jogging	12
Swimming fast	10
Cycling, tennis	7
Sitting	1

Apart from just sitting, these are all sustained exercise and you will be able to keep going for only a limited length of time before you have to stop and rest and finally call a halt altogether. The benefit of brisk walking is that you can sustain it for a considerably longer period of time. If possible walk into work each day.

To walk one mile (half an hour of time) will burn up about 150 calories. Cycling the same distance, 10 minutes plus stops at traffic lights, only 70 calories.

Burning off calories

Here are some favourite foods with their calorie values and the time it would take to burn off those calories by brisk walking.

If you need to burn up about 200 calories you must walk briskly for ¾ hour. If you need to burn up about 400 calories you must walk briskly for 1½ hours. This equals one Mars bar! Soft drinks are full of calories with little or no nutritional value. Also, they contain sodium which causes your body to retain fluid, therefore increasing your body weight and adding inches.

Foods	Calorie Value	Walking time to burn them up
2 slices toast with butter and marmalade	370	1 hour 14 minutes
Cream cheese and biscuits	350	1 hour 10 minutes
1 chocolate Yorkie bar 50 g/2 oz	330	1 hour 7 minutes
1 corned beef sandwich	326	1 hour 5 minutes
1 packet peanuts 50 g/2 oz	320	1 hour 4 minutes
1 packet crisps 50 g/2 oz	318	1 hour 3 minutes
1 piece chocolate cake	282	56 minutes

Foods	Calorie Value	Walking time to burn them up
1 sausage roll	268	54 minutes
1 glass beer (600 ml/1 pint)	180	36 minutes
1 cup cocoa	152	30 minutes
1 ice cream 75 g/3 oz	112	24 minutes

Chapter 5

Shape where you want it: EXERCISE

*T*he principle of balance you apply to your eating habits must also apply to exercise. Fanatical concentration and effort with exercising whether it is to shape, tone, reduce, build-up or strengthen is as out of balance as fanatical dieting. You become obsessed and single-minded to the point of imbalance to yourself and boredom to others.

Why exercise?

Exercise is essential to keep you healthy and fit; to allow you to be as supple and free as possible in your movements, for the rest of your life; to prevent you from becoming overweight or out of shape. But what is health and fitness?

Health is the absence of disease.

Fitness is the possession of strength, stamina and suppleness.

The definitions need be only this simple. And the simpler the definitions are kept, the easier the understanding of health or fitness. But we tend to qualify them and say 'My health is not very good' or 'I am not as fit as I should be or need to be'. So immediately we are applying our individual requirements for the lifestyle that we lead and the things that we wish to do, for which we need either 'better health' or a 'higher standard of fitness'. The World Health Organisation states, 'Health is a state of complete physical, mental and social well-being and not merely the absence of disease or infirmity.' The Office of Health Economics states, 'A person should be regarded as healthy provided he can remain socially and economically active, even though he may have to suffer some health disability or discomfort.'

Similarly, fitness is further qualified as being in a suitable condition to fulfil your mental and physical requirements competently, upon demand. How fit should you be? As fit as your lifestyle requires *plus* a little more so that your on-going activities are coped with easily and unexpected demands can be met without undue stress; your *potential*, of strength, stamina and suppleness, should always be there; the fitter you are the more you can do.

The simple, short definitions above are apt; adapt yourself to them.

Metabolism

Metabolism, briefly, is a series of chemical changes that take place in your body in order to maintain life; the tissues are continuously being broken down (by wear and tear) and re-built. Your *basic* metabolism is the minimum amount of energy used by your body, at rest, to maintain your life, and your metabolic *rate* is the expression of this energy in terms of calories, provided by the food you eat, which is then converted into energy.

If you divide your calorie intake, and therefore your energy, into sixths, just over half of the total is used up by your natural process of being alive including your physical and mental activity. About another sixth is

Your metabolic rate determines the rate at which your body uses its intake of calories. You should only eat what your body needs. If you eat too much, the calories are stored as fat.

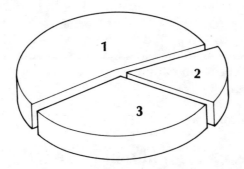

1. ENERGY (calories)
required in normal daily living to build tissues and repair tissues, for muscle movement and all bodily functions
Just over ½

2. ENERGY (calories)
required to provide bodily warmth
About ¹/₆

3. EXCESS ENERGY (calories)
stored as fat (also creating an extra burden on the heart)
About ⅓!
SO eat less, use it up by exercising or both

converted into keeping you warm. The remainder, about one-third of the total, quite a high percentage, is often excess and converted into fat, and stored as such! For this to happen, perhaps you are eating too much or exercising too little, or both.

Exercise stops you from getting sluggish, both physically and mentally. Mental sluggishness may be *caused* by physical sluggishness and vice versa. This is because the mind and the body cannot be divorced one from the other and what affects one affects both, whether beneficially or adversely. When you feel mentally slow, especially first thing in the morning, a quick bout of exercise in the fresh air can often clear an inert, stale attitude of mind. Your disciplined effort can break that mental pattern. It's rather like being in a hot, airless room for too long and becoming unpleasantly inert; when you open the window and let in the fresh air, which activates the room's atmosphere, you liven up, 'blow the cobwebs away'.

Exercise, the right exercise, can arouse a slow metabolism.

Why exercise and diet go together

Each day's food intake need only be enough to provide energy to build and repair your tissues, energy to activate you and energy for your sufficient warmth. To become slimmer or lighter in weight, the remaining one-third of energy must not be allowed to accrue and this can be achieved by either regular exercise or by eating less, so that there is no excess to be carried around by your body in the shape of unrequired, ungainly fat (also putting an unnecessary or harmful workload on to your heart and lungs). Or you can do both: exercise more and eat less, when results both visual and in terms of well-being will be apparent more quickly. Eating less has already been discussed. Here, we are concerned with appropriate, safe exercising.

The meaning of 'aerobic'

Aerobic means 'with oxygen'. The other direct source of energy (apart from food/calorie intake) is the oxygen you breathe in. Aerobics is a general term given to a manner of exercising, often to music; and you may have attended an aerobics dance class, its aim being to improve the functioning of the heart and circulation with the benefits that will then result. It can be quite a strenuous routine, even when commenced at low-level, and suits the minority rather than the majority.

But aerobic functioning is an ongoing process throughout your life: your oxygen intake is converted to produce a high-energy compound, which energy you expend during physical activity of any sort. Your bloodstream transports this supply to all your muscles, so the better your intake and supply of oxygen (i.e. your breathing ability) and the performance of your heart and circulatory system, the more physically effective you will be. This is called your aerobic *capacity*.

At the moment, perhaps you experience difficulty or stress in certain daily activities: walking up hills, climbing upstairs, walking long distances or even short ones, running – you get out of breath, or tired, or just 'haven't got the energy'. If you can increase your aerobic capacity and physical performance to a level greater than that which you actually require for your daily living, then any activity using less than your capacity becomes easy, effortless and a pleasure – because you can do it! This will of course benefit your mind and life in general will become easier, less strained and more enjoyable. And because your potential is good, any sudden demand in excess of your daily requirement can be met, not necessarily without effort but certainly without detriment.

Choice of exercise

It is important to choose the right sort of exercise for the individual that you are. You do not have to attend an aerobics class to achieve results. Think of exercise less in terms of exercise-for-fitness-sake and more for your enjoyment! Choose a form of exercise or sport or game that suits you and start it at a low level of effort and increase as you feel comfortably able. Take instruction!

The benefits whether of improvement in your aerobic capacity or in terms of toning and shaping will follow naturally.

Swimming is the best overall exercise because you use your entire body, you need your breathing to be good and you can sustain this overall exercise more easily and for longer because your body is less weighted by gravity due to the bouyancy of the water. Dancing is also an excellent overall exercise, as is table-tennis. More strenuous are tennis, badminton and squash; but if you are older and these are new or renewed forms of exercise consult your GP first – any sustained exercising like these make a tremendous demand on a system which is not prepared or used to it.

Walking and cycling are also excellent. If you are accustomed to neither, start for short distances, increasing as you feel able until perhaps you are walking or cycling to and from work. If you don't already, you may come to enjoy it!

You also have to recognise which forms of exercise really do not suit you, according to your age, physical structure and natural, individual capability and make-up. For example, you may rule out swimming simply because you don't like getting wet! A very human reason. Racket-and-ball games, for example, also require concentration and good co-ordination of your eye, racket, ball, and a partner and a court to play on.

Sustained exercise

Much has been said about sustained exercise and its benefits and dangers, with particular reference to jogging and aerobics. But any exercise is sustained if you continue it for any length of time without stopping; whether it is walking, dancing, cycling, swimming, jogging, aerobics or a gym routine. When you reach the point of needing to stop because your reactions are becoming uncomfortable or even distressing, you should be able to do so. Not to do so is the point at which sustained exercise becomes potentially dangerous.

The danger signals are: getting badly out of breath, becoming unpleasantly tired, your muscles beginning to shake (if you continue they may go into spasm or even 'seize up on you' which is nature's way of making you stop), and being aware of your heart pumping uncomfortably and the blood pounding in your ears. Your system is warning you and you must listen to it.

If you continue to suffer because of your reactions you will have to accept that this one or that one is not for you – and find an alternative form of exercise which you can learn to sustain with success and enjoyment.

The only way to shape

General exercise always helps you to slim but may not shape you where you want. The only way to shape in specific areas is with specific exercise. The warm-up sequence has been designed to achieve just this, as has the gym routine.

If you have a sluggish system this kind of all-over exercise is a MUST. You must bend and stretch and then bend and stretch again, and again. Waking up your metabolism may get the slimming process started for you better than any other way. Toned-up muscles also take up less space so you will begin to measure less, your body will become firmer and you will look more attractive. Accompany this with a slim-orientated diet and you shouldn't fail. Dietary methods on their own can be hit and miss. How often have you said, or overheard someone say, 'I have been eating differently but it never comes off in the right place'.

This is where the specifically devised exercises in this book will help you. They are designed to tone, slim and shape you – and you can be selective, leaving out some of the movements or increasing others to suit your personal requirements.

The warm-up sequence is free standing, simple, and can be done each day. It will benefit you overall and help shape you generally and in specific areas.

The gym routine, using equipment in your local multi-gym, will also benefit you overall. It is an extension of the warm-up sequence movements but by using the equipment your muscles are working against the resistance of weights. Provided you use each piece correctly the benefit will be more specific and quicker and it is the most effective way to control your shape where you want it.

Individual, not competitive

Neither of these methods of exercise is competitive.

Some people thrive on physical competition, games or sports, where others are hopeless for a variety of very human reasons: the extra exertion required to be part of a team, or playing in opposition, may be that fraction too much. You might experience a sense of failure or guilt because of this. Or you just may not be as socially inclined as some activities require of you. There can also be a danger element for some of you if you attempt to exercise or 're-shape' on a competitive basis. For example, working out with a time-limit set by the clock, or by moving to a definite beat of pre-recorded music, or by trying to keep up with the rest of the class, especially if the others are much younger than you. For an older woman, the very individual approach offered in this book can be great comfort and give confidence. And if you are fortunate enough to join a class where the instruction follows the methods set out in this book, you can be a 66-year-old among 16 year-olds and not feel out of place. Your energy output may be more reserved but your staying power will possibly outshine them (one of the privileges of growing older!). This form of exercising really is for all ages.

Competition, of course, is not bad – far from it – it can

be great fun, a good stimulus and an education in relationships. Some people thrive on it. But you can be, whatever your age, overwhelmed by a possible element of competition in a field in which you may not feel very confident at any rate. And then you just stop going to your club or class. By taking away that competitive element, for those who are not easy with it, individual success not only stands a chance but can almost be guaranteed.

Safety

Your individual approach can be as strenuous as you feel comfortable with and, as you learn to be your own judge of your initial capability and potential, you will always carry with you the necessary element of safety. You must become your own best judge of what you can do and cannot do. If you listen to the way you respond to these exercises you cannot overdo it. Always start at the lowest contribution of effort and increase your effort gradually, only as you acquire greater ability to do so. Listen to your own system. You have to take responsibility for yourself and if you are not sure you must consult your GP. And you must certainly consult him if you, or your family, have a history of heart, circulatory or other medical or structural problems.

Specific precautions and 'do's and don'ts' are listed at the start of both the warm-up sequence and the gym routine.

Pulse rate

Your *pulse* is the impulse of your blood as it is transmitted by the muscle contraction of your heart (from the left ventricle) to your arteries (and thence around your body).

Your *pulse rate* is the number of impulses, or beats, that occur per minute. The normal, average rate for an adult is approximately 70 impulses per minute.

Physical activity, illness, stress or distress (whether physical, mental or emotional) will alter this rate. In the case of physical activity your pulse rate will increase.

There is a maximum level above which you should not exercise for safety's sake.

In modern fitness centres which have been specifically designed for physical effort with gymnasia their centre of attaction, it is now possible to undergo a very thorough mechanical and electrical testing of the physical demand in which you may safely indulge, together with an assessment of your natural potential. But this can be costly and is perhaps also for the dedicated enthusiast of fitness who may then be given quite a strenuous work-out which is supervised and monitored. Pulse rate would be one of the safety measures to be checked.

For everyday health and shaping, and for the woman exercising at home or in her local gym, this is not necessary. Your capacity and potential can be assessed quite simply and easily by yourself. First, by being aware of your reactions to types and degrees of exercise and taking personal responsibility and second, by checking your pulse rate very simply, by hand.

Resting Pulse Rate First, feel for the pulse of your radial artery at your wrist (on the thumb-side: this is where a GP or nurse would check it), or of the carotid artery at the side of your neck. Use your middle or ring finger to do this because your thumb and forefinger have quite a strong beat of their own and this could confuse you. With a stop-watch, or better still with somebody timing you, for a period of 6 seconds count the number of times that you feel the pulse beat (say, 7). Multiply this figure by 10 (70) and you will have the number of times that your resting pulse beats per minute.

Safety Level Maximum From the number 200, subtract the number of decades that you have age (e.g. if you are 30, deduct 30 = 170; if you are 38 or 42, deduct 40 = 160). This is the maximum number of times that your pulse may beat safely when you are working your body hard.

Working Pulse Rate While exercising, find your pulse rate by the same method as for the resting pulse rate, but the figure you arrive at will be higher, perhaps much higher, because you have just been, or still are, very active. This is your working pulse rate and should never exceed your safety level maximum.

If your working pulse rate becomes too close to your safety level maximum you must stop and rest, however fit and able you feel and despite not necessarily experiencing any other 'danger signals'.

The difference between bodyshaping and body-building

When you exercise, your muscles must tone up, begin to lose fat and therefore change their shape.

When your exercising is light and against minimum resistance, as you increase your speed to fairly fast your muscles will tighten and should, with time, decrease in measurement. Some people may realise dramatic results, for others it will take longer. Changing your eating habits will speed up the process even more. This is *bodyshaping*. It is within the natural, safe capability of most people.

Body building is similar exercising but done more slowly to a much greater resistance of weights on the gym equipment. Your muscles are being worked so hard that they develop and the measurement will increase.

When you fully understand what you are doing, and why, you can combine the two if necessary. For example, if you are thin in one area (say, calves or chest) you will be able to body build in that area and body shape everywhere else.

Breathing

A lot of emphasis is put on 'abdominal breathing', in other words being conscious of using your abdomen, sometimes to the point of exaggeration, as you breathe.

If you are healthy, albeit perhaps not very fit, you will be using your abdominal muscles as you breathe: you can't help it, because in the process of normal respiration your abdominal muscles play a major role.

The important thing is not to be conscious of what is happening, but to have the muscles of your abdomen and those of your rib cage in the best possible condition, well-toned and capable of relaxing, enabling your lungs to enlarge to maximum capacity and fill deeply with air, and then by the relaxation of these muscles expel it. (Breathing *out* fully is very important to get rid of carbon dioxide waste.) This is what ensures that your process of breathing is correct and effective, a natural process that requires no conscious thought or monitoring.

Your abdominal and rib cage muscles are exercised and toned in your warm-up sequence and gym routine.

Relaxation

Rest after any sustained activity, whether it is physical or mental (and let this include after the effort of your daily nine to five occupation). It is not a sign of weakness but a sign of common sense and awareness, wisdom and maturity. If the family screams at you for attention, make them wait! Self-respect on your part can only benefit you and you will perhaps give them a greater sense of consideration and self-discipline.

A few moments alone, quietly, lying on the floor after exercise or when you get home from work, works wonders! It doesn't matter what age you are, young or old, it's a good, balanced habit. The benefits are invaluable. Try it!

Your target!

Don't set an unrealistic target. To be fit has become a craze recently as, for some women, has excessive thinness. We are all made basically the same way but over the years due to the environment, circumstances, occupation, child-bearing, hobbies, stresses (physical, mental and emotional) we develop individually and this affects the way we use, and can use, our physical body. This needs to be taken into account so that you can set yourself a realistic target to re-shape yourself.

There is no need to be bone-thin. It may be the fashion but it is rarely pretty and a few soft curves are a woman's natural body shape and appeal.

Also, there is a level for you as an individual, in your shape and weight, at which you will feel happy. Go below this level and you may begin to feel distressed in some way: fatigued, without energy, irritable, miserable. The common comparison of height, age and weight is not really applicable. When you can say: 'I feel good at this shape and weight, it suits me, I'm happy like this' – then that's the level to work to, and stop there.

Before you begin

Starting and ending your exercise routine

Your physical performance will be better if your breathing performance is good. Start each exercise session, whether you are spending 10 minutes daily at home (warm-up sequence) or a session in the gym (warm-up sequence followed by gym routine) standing, if possible by an open window, breathing deeply. Just a few times is enough to prepare your body for the ensuing demands.

End each exercise session lying on the floor on your back, relaxing. Give your lungs, heart and muscles, which have just been working, a chance to rest. Stay there until your breathing and heart beat have resumed a natural, quiet rhythm. It will only take a few minutes.

The importance of good breathing and effective relaxation cannot be emphasised too much.

Sets and repetitions

Perform each exercise to the right side and to the left side (where applicable), say 5 times: this is 1 SET of 5 REPETITIONS (1x5).

Repeat this 3 times: this is 3 SETS of 5 REPETITIONS (3x5).

So a SET is made up of the *same* exercise repeated a given number of times.

Perform the required number of sets and then move on to the next exercise or piece of gym equipment, and follow exactly the same method, that is, complete your work with one exercise or at one piece of equipment and don't return to it.

While doing the gym routine, rest between sets at the chosen equipment. This gives you a balance of exercise/rest/exercise/rest, producing a more effective and sustainable peformance. Gradually increase the number of repetitions within a set (e.g. 3x5, 3x7, 3x9) or the number of sets (e.g. 3x5, 4x5, 5x5) if you want to, but with regular gymnasium exercising this is not necessary. Overdoing it will bring you to body building rather than body shaping. It will also take more time when time may be at a premium.

Isometrics

Stop an exercise at the level where you feel the appropriate muscles are working their hardest and hold this position for *7 seconds only*. This is working your muscles *isometrically*. Isometric exercise is effective but very powerful and should be done, per exercise, *once daily only*.

Breathlessness during warm-up sequence and gym routine

You will find yourself out of breath during some of the execises. This may be due not only to the effort you are putting into it but also to the position you have taken up. In the exercises in which your arms are raised, your rib cage cannot expand and relax so your breathing pattern has to alter. It is good to be out of breath during exercising. This proves that your lungs and heart are being exercised as well as your muscles and joints, and your aerobic capacity will improve.

Each exercise is explained as follows

- With a diagram.
- Why you are doing it (i.e. for which part of your body).
- The number of sets and repetitions.
- How you do it.
- Extending it: some of the exercises can be extended for greater benefit, once you are fluent with them. The way to extend them is given at the end of each description, where appropriate.

SP = Starting position; **R** = Right; **L** = Left.

Chapter 6

THE WARM-UP SEQUENCE

*T*he complete warm-up sequence will shape and slim you if practised daily. It improves your circulation, mobilises your joints and strengthens and tones your muscles. It will also improve your posture and walking pattern, both of which help to shape you.

The warm-up sequence is also an essential introduction for your body before going on to more demanding equipment. It is *part of* your gym routine.

It is effective as a sequence on its own. Practised daily, and together with a suitable diet, you will soon have the results even if you choose not to follow it with the gym routine (although the latter will benefit you in specific areas that much more quickly).

It won't take you long to grasp and remember the exercises and then each movement will follow on smoothly from the last and you can complete the entire sequence as one continuous movement.

Do's and don'ts

1. DO keep your meals light and small, or non-existent before warm-up sequence.

2. DO the warm-up sequence daily if you want results. It will only take you about 10 to 15 minutes. To begin with, do each exercise once and gradually increase to the maximum number of sets and repetitions shown at each exercise/diagram. As you become familiar with it, speed it up and put more zest and effort into it. This is more effective than repeating the sequence.

3. DO try it without shoes: you will learn to mould your bare feet to the floor. This will increase your sensitivity and sense of physical balance and you can also exercise your feet, toes and ankles more effectively without shoes.

4. DO hold on to something (back of chair, door handle, table top) to steady yourself, if necessary, until in due course you can exercise completely free-standing. Each exercise is designed to benefit a specific area and if to begin with you have difficulty in keeping your body straight when required to do so you may tend to compensate by tipping to one side or straining, so that you are not exercising the appropriate areas really effectively. For the same reasons you could also, to begin with, do exercises 2, 3, 4, 5, 6 sitting in an upright chair.

5. DO exercise your abdominal muscles last. In the warm-up sequence you are, intentionally, working from top-to-toe. All exercises specifically for the abdomen are powerful and quite tiring. For this reason you always do these last.

6. DO protect your spine. When you are exercising on your back you must protect your spine. The very irregularity in shape and size and the extreme solid boniness of your vertebrae indicates just how vitally your nervous system needs to be protected. Even with this protection your spine is incredibly sensitive and it needs a buffer between it and the inanimate insensitivity of all floors. Exercises where you are working with your back and head in contact with the floor *must* be done on a carpet-type floor covering which will not slip as you move. Always press your back flat against the floor, if possible, before attempting abdominal exercises.

7. NEVER work through pain. Pain is warning you that something is wrong and you must stop and rest, or perhaps seek medical help.

8. DON'T exercise if you are pregnant or have a history of high-blood pressure, heart irregularities or other medical or structural problems, without consulting your GP first.

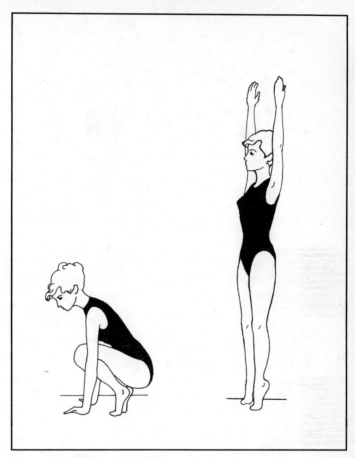

1   Overall stretch   x1

SP   Squat close to floor, feet together, on tip-toe.

Slowly straighten up, still on tip-toe, and stretch upwards, raising your arms to keep your balance as you tense your muscles, and stretch up from your toes to the top of your head: feet, ankles, calves, front and back of thighs, buttocks, abdomen, waist, chest, shoulders, neck, arms right up to finger tips. Balance for a moment. 'Collapse' and relax to SP.

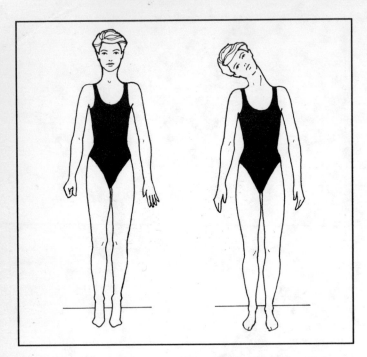

2   Extremities: *feet/hands/neck/shoulders*
x5 each

SP   Stand, feet together or slightly apart.

1.   Rise up and down on your toes.
2.   Clench and stretch your fingers.
3.   From the wrist, shake relaxed hands up and down, side to side, circle in one direction then the other.
4.   Gently tip head to R and then to L.
5.   Slowly and smoothly drop your head forward to your chest then straighten up your neck. Drop your head back, then straighten up your neck. Turn head to R, forward, to L, forward again. (Do each movement in 5 just once.)
6.   Shrug your shoulders, up and down; circle them round and round, slowly then quickly.

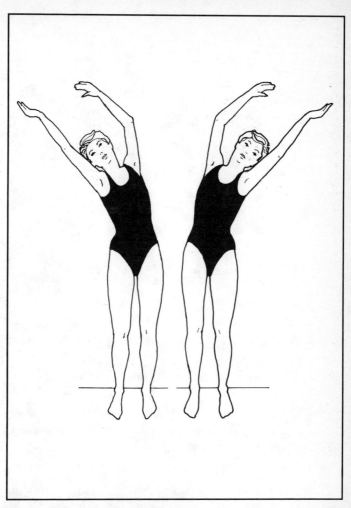

3   Side of body, waist   x3

SP   Stand with feet apart and raise arms straight up.

Keeping your arms straight, raise up at the waist and
from your waist drop your body sideways to the right,
straighten up and then drop sideways to the left. Keep
your feet flat on the ground throughout.

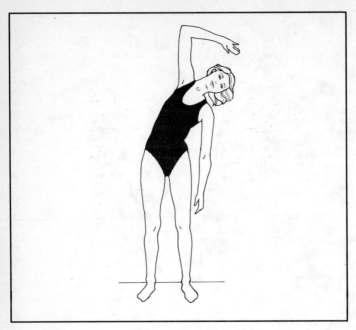

4   Ribcage, side of body, waist   3x5

SP   Stand with feet apart, body facing to front, arms by your side.

Raise R arm curved over your head, raise up at waist, drop body to L from waist. Then bounce from waist to L side 5 times. Relax to SP. Reverse sides.

This forms 1 set of 5 repetitions (1x5).

As you stretch your top arm over your head, 'lead' with your little finger; this ensures that you keep your *palm upwards,* and exercise the required muscles. (Try otherwise and you will feel the difference.)

To extend Stretch the arm down by your side, be aware of the position of your finger tips against your leg. When you drop to that side with each bounce aim to reach a little further down that leg. You will feel the increased stretch on the other side of your body.

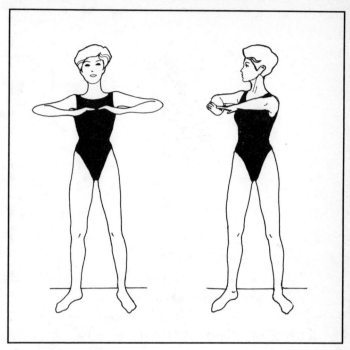

5   Waist   3x5

SP   Stand with feet apart, body facing to front. Bend elbows, arms across chest, finger tips touching.

Raise up at waist and from your waist twist top of body to R. Try to keep your hips facing to the front. Five little bouncy movements stretching you to the R. Relax to SP. Reverse sides. This forms 1 set of 5 repetitions (1x5).

To extend After you have twisted to the side, 'mark' the position of your back elbow in relation to the wall behind you. With each bounce see how far round that elbow moves from the first position you 'marked'. But, remember to keep your arms in their original position across your chest, your hips to the front and your waist raised up. If you can do this, it's a really effective exercise for your waist.

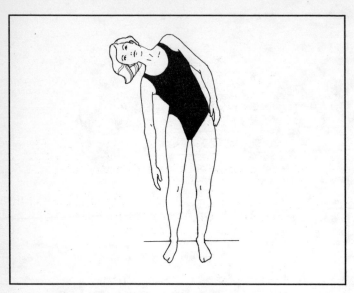

6   Waist and hips at side   3x5

SP   Stand with feet apart, body facing to front, arms by
your sides.

Raise up at waist and from your waist drop to R as far as
you can. Five little bouncy movements stretching you
downwards to the R. Relax to SP. Reverse sides.
This forms 1 set of 5 repetitions (1x5).

To extend Be aware of the position of your fingers
against your leg when you drop to the side. With each
bounce aim to reach a little further down that leg. The
other side of your body will be really stretched.

7   Waist, abdomen, spine   3 sets

SP   Stand with feet apart, body facing to front, arms up
in the air.

Raise up at waist, bend knees to maintain balance, arch
body backwards. Five bouncy movements backwards.

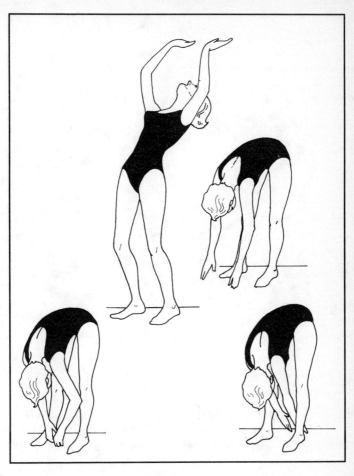

Straighten, keeping raised at waist, then drop forward, straightening legs, bounce (with large reflex), hands touching floor once in front of feet, once between feet, once through feet. Relax to SP.
This forms 1 set.

To extend After you have arched backwards, visualise the position of your fingers against the wall behind you. With each bounce backwards see how far back your finger tips 'measure'.

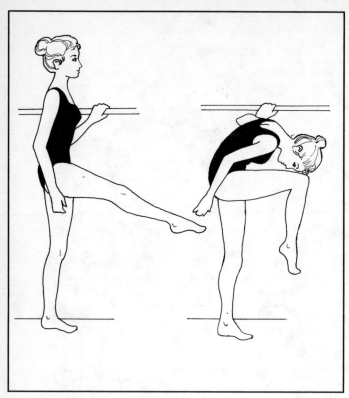

8 Abdomen, spine   3 sets

SP Stand with feet together. Hold on to something if
necessary for balance.

Raise R leg, bent at the knee, swing backwards and
forwards from the hip once. Then straighten leg and
swing backwards and forwards from the hip once. Repeat
with L leg.
This forms 1 set.

To extend Balance on L leg, bend R knee up and curl
spine over until forehead touches bent knee. Relax to SP.
Reverse sides.
This forms 1 set.

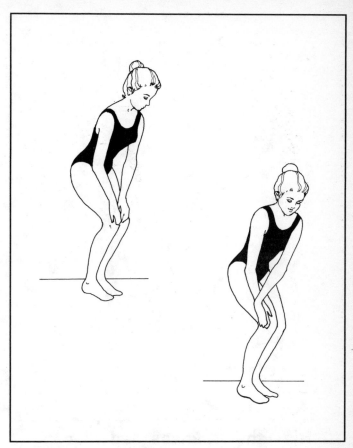

9   Hips, low spine, knees   x1

SP   Stand, feet together, knees bent, hands on knees.

Circle knees to R, 5 times, to L, 5 times. Place both hands to R side of bent knees, push knees gently to L, 5 times. Change hands to L side, push knees gently to R, 5 times. Relax to SP.

You should feel the effect mostly in your hip, knee and ankle joints. Keep soles of feet flat on the floor throughout.

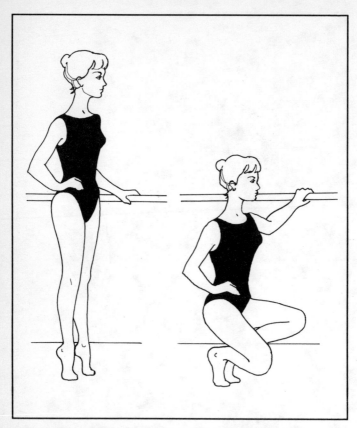

10 Hips, thighs, knees, abdomen

x5 each position

**DON'T DO THIS EXERCISE IF YOUR KNEES
TROUBLE YOU IN ANY WAY.**

SP   a) Stand with feet angled at 10 to 2, i.e. heels
together, toes apart.

SP   b) Stand with feet together at 'mid-day', i.e. heels
and toes together.

Deep knee bend, straighten up, 5 times. Relax to
SP.

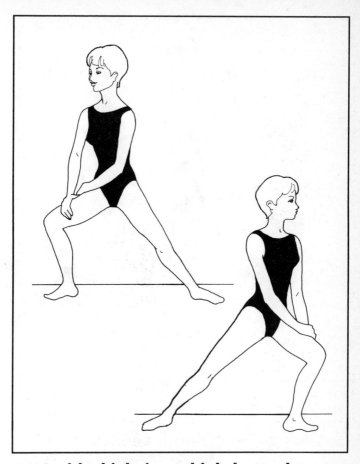

11 Inside thigh, front thigh, buttocks 3x3

SP Take up position as in diagram. Stride, with R front leg bent, L back leg straight. Turn out your L hip, back foot facing backwards, keep soles of both feet entirely on floor.

Lunge forwards over front bent leg, 5 times, keeping trunk of body upright as you lunge. Relax to SP. Reverse sides.

This forms 1 set of 3 repetitions (1x3).

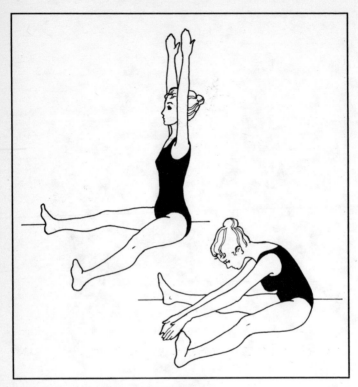

12 Low spine, abdomen   3x5

SP   Sit on floor, feet apart, legs straight.

Raise arms in air. Raise up at waist, stretch up and
forwards from your low spine until fingers touch the
floor between your feet. Five little stretch movements
and as you stretch forwards touch the floor further off
each time. Relax to SP.
This forms 1 set of 5 repetitions (1x5).

You should feel the stretch in your low spine. This
exercise will also 'squeeze' the contents of your abdomen
as you bounce over it and forwards, very beneficial if you
suffer from constipation. The stretch is from your low
spine and not your arm sockets!

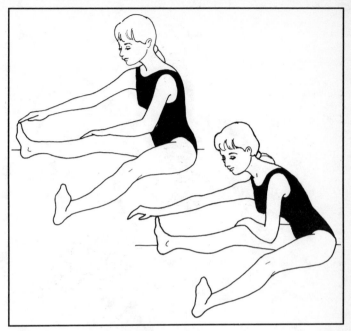

13 Low spine, waist, hips, knees   3x5

SP   Sit on floor, feet apart, legs straight, toes up in the air.

Place L hand on R knee, to help keep that leg straight. Stretch your R hand to touch R toes. Five bouncy movements, touching your toes with
1) your finger tips
2) finger middle joints
3) knuckle joints
4) palm of hand
5) heel of hand
Relax to SP. Reverse sides.
This forms 1 set of 5 repetitions (1x5). The stretch is from your low spine and not your arm sockets!

To extend Point your toes away from you as you do the exercise. Your low spine has to stretch further.

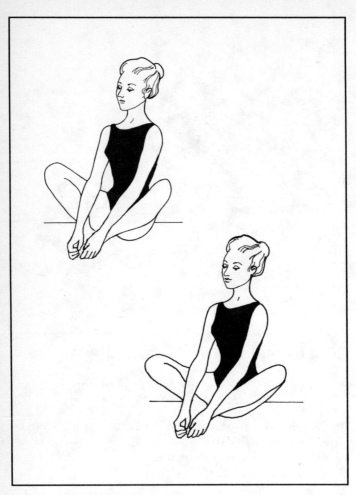

14 Inside thigh at top x5

SP Sit on floor, soles of feet touching, feet quite close to your body, knees bent and up in the air. Clasp your toes with your hands to steady your body.

Keeping your feet still, move knees down towards the floor. Five times, but on the last movement, hold isometrically. Relax to SP.

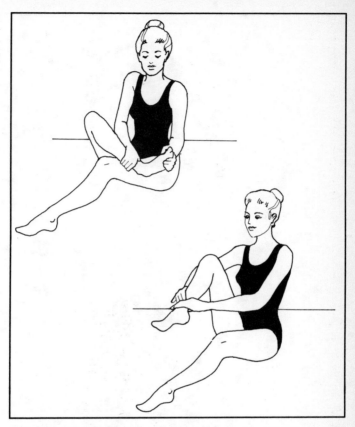

15 Ankle joints   x5 each side

SP   Sit on floor, legs straight.

Place R foot across L knee. With R hand, hold just above R ankle joint then grasp R toes with L hand, as in diagram. Using L hand to do the work of moving your foot (i.e. passive movement) circle foot 5 times in each direction. If you slightly bend the underneath leg this will give clearance from the floor to give you enough space to make a good circling movement. Then, with both hands grasp just above R ankle and shake foot, 5 times. Relax to SP. Reverse sides.

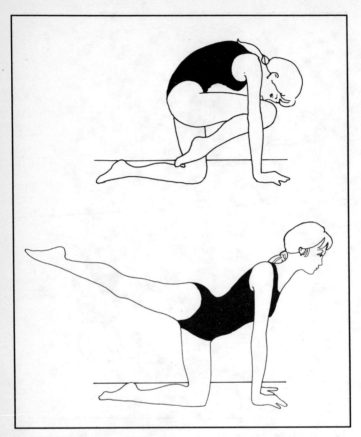

16 Hips, low back   3 sets

SP Cat-crouch, i.e. kneel on all fours.

Curling your spine, bring R knee to forehead, then
stretch same leg out behind you, arching spine, head up.
Relax to SP. Reverse sides.
This forms 1 set.

To extend After you have stretched your leg out behind
you, stretch it as far back and *up* as you can, from the *hip*.
Do this just once, each side, because this is a powerful
movement.

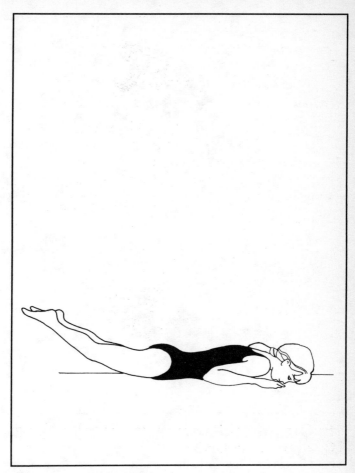

17 Low back, back of thighs at top

x5 each side

SP On carpet, lie full length on your tummy, elbows bent, hands at shoulder level, elbows on floor.

Keep legs straight and raise them up from the floor. Keep hips on floor. 5 times. Relax to SP.

To extend Hold the 5th time isometrically, if you can!

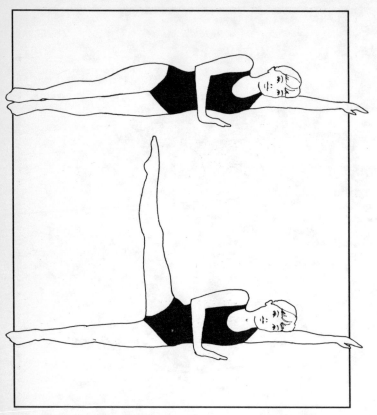

18 Outside thighs   x5 each side

SP   On carpet, lie on L side, body and legs in straight
line, with your head resting on a straight L arm.

Kick R leg up sideways, keeping leg and body straight.
Lower leg to SP, 5 times. Roll over and reverse side, 5
times.

To extend Lower leg as slowly as possible. Gravity is
taking that leg down. To counteract gravity, if you control
the speed down you will have to work your outside thigh
muscles, not only in raising your leg but also in lowering
it.

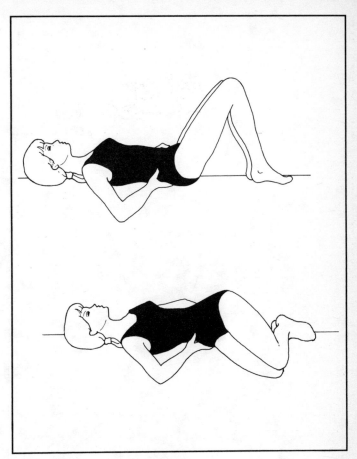

19 Waist, hips, thighs   5 sets

SP   On carpet, lie on back, bend knees, keep feet on
      floor. Keep hands on hips, thumbs upwards.

Swing legs over to R until knees touch floor. Keep knees
together and feet, R hip and shoulders in contact with
floor. Return to SP. Swing over to L side until knees touch
floor keeping knees together and feet, L hip and
shoulders in contact with floor. Return to SP.
This forms 1 set.

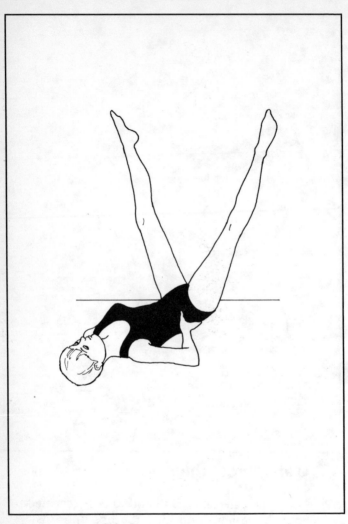

20 Inside thigh   x5

SP   On carpet, lie on back, raise straight legs in the air,
hands on your hips (thumbs upwards) for balance.

Open legs very slowly, as wide as possible, then close
together very slowly.

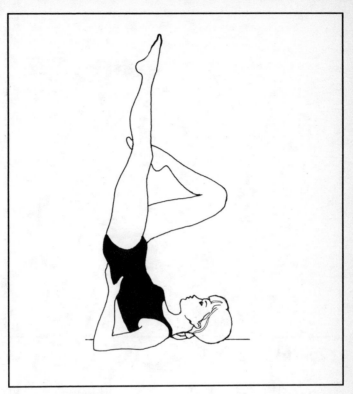

21 Hips, knees x5

DON'T DO THIS ONE IF YOU HAVE HIGH BLOOD PRESSURE.

SP On carpet, lie on your back.

Take up position as in diagram: shoulder-stand, supporting yourself at your hips with your hands. 'Cycle' your legs in the air, several times.
Relax to SP.

Take care as you come down, gently to *curl* your spine down. Roll down with knees bent and a rounded back. This protects your spine from too fierce a contact with the floor on the way down.

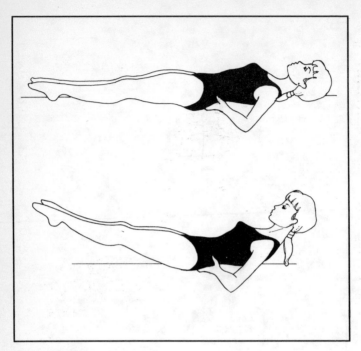

22 Abdomen   x5

SP   On carpet, lie flat on back, legs straight, hands on your hips for balance. Flatten your spine against the floor.

Raise straight legs and head at the same time, equal in distance from floor, until you can just see your feet. Relax to SP. 5 times but on the 5th time hold isometrically.

You should feel your abdominal muscles pulling low down. This position will also exercise your abdominal muscles higher up, just below your diaphragm area, but you may feel this less.

Raising straight legs like this is a strong abdominal exercise and if you have a 'hollow back' it may be too uncomfortable and you will be wise not to do it. You can try the same exercise with bent knees.

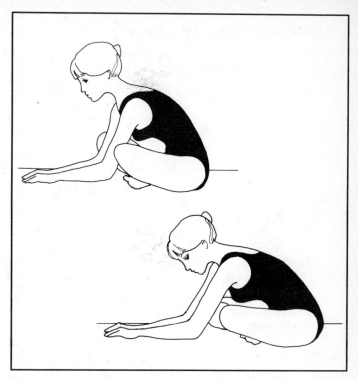

23 To ease low spine after doing 22   x1

SP On carpet, as you sit up after doing exercise 22, sit into cross-legged position.

Lean your body forwards over your crossed legs. Place your elbows, forearms and hands on the floor in front of you. Stretching forwards from low spine, push your hands as far forwards on the floor as you can, *keeping your bottom, elbows and forearms on floor.*

This is an excellent exercise to take ache or strain out of your low spine area. The stretch is from your low spine and not your arm sockets!

NOW LIE FLAT ON FLOOR, ON YOUR BACK, FOR A FEW MINUTES AND COMPLETELY *RELAX*.

Flattening your abdomen

If you have a plump tummy just because you eat too much and have become fat, there is no better way of reducing your abdomen than by adhering to one of the slimming diets described on pages 63 to 67. This will help you cope with your excess fat but, as you know, it won't necessarily give you the shape where you want it. Only by combining your slimming diet with specific exercising will you achieve this. It is more difficult however for those of you who have lost your tummy shape after having children, and also for older women, because you may have not exercised properly for some years.

If over the years you have let this area go and not kept yourself in trim, the lack of tone in these very important abdominal muscles allows them to sag and bulge because you have no bony structure in the front of you to prevent this from happening. The soft organs within you, which these muscles should be protecting and keeping in position, are displaced by the pull of gravity. It is well worth concentrating on exercising your tummy and the following exercises, additional to the warm-up sequence and gym routine, can be done regularly at home.

Exercise one

SP On carpet, lie on your back, on the floor, with straight legs.

Breathe in and raise your straight R leg. Breath out and lower it. Do the same with your L leg. Do this several times. Then breathe in and raise your R leg, and as you breathe out lower it but cross it over your L leg. Breathe in, raise your R leg again and as you breathe out lower it to SP. Do the same with your left leg. Do this several times.

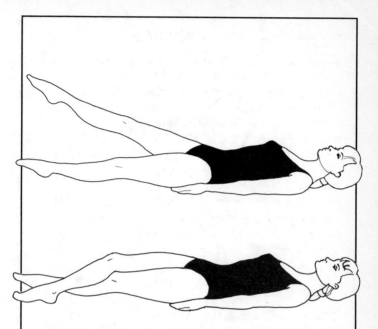

This exercises your very low abdominal muscles. You can extend this exercise by raising both straight legs together as you breathe in, breathing out as you lower them. Always stop at the level at which you feel your low abdominal muscles working their hardest. If this exercise gives you discomfort in your low back, place your hands on your hips, thumbs uppermost, to give your low trunk support. If this does not ease your lower back, leave out this exercise.

Exercise two

SP   On carpet, lie on your back, on the floor, with your knees bent.

Tighten your abdominal muscles so that your tummy pulls in and your back flattens to the floor. Relax. Do this several times and the last time hold isometrically.

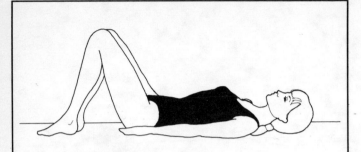

Get into the habit of pulling in your tummy muscles throughout the day, as you wash up or watch the television. Make a rule with yourself to walk upstairs with them pulled in, and the same on the way down again.

Exercise three

This is the 'bum-walk'!

SP On carpet, sit on the floor with your legs straight out, your hands resting lightly on top of your thighs and your back as straight as possible.

Pull in your tummy muscles and 'walk' forward on your buttocks, right, left, right, left until you have crossed the room this way. As you get good at it, try it backwards! It will help to reduce your bottom as well!

Toning your tummy.

Always pull your tummy in when you lift or move heavy or cumbersome objects.

Did you have low backache during your pregnancy? There is a definite connection between this and a tummy that afterwards just will not return to shape. The internal oblique and transverse abdominal muscles originate on your low spine and as they stretch and 'give' during pregnancy many women experience severe pain at these points of origin. These

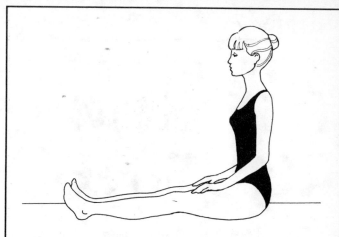

muscles contract in due course after childbirth, especially if you have breastfed your baby, but it is often women who have experienced severe pain during pregnancy who have most difficulty in regaining their abdominal shape. Warm-up sequence and gym routine will help, and so will the above additional exercises and all exercises that ease your low spine. If you are immediately post-natal you should *never* exercise without the approval of your doctor, midwife or physiotherapist. But if your pregnancy or childbirth is well behind you, try the above exercises. Breast-feeding will help to re-shape your abdomen.

Alas, it does not take actual childbirth to give this unwanted tone-less tummy. Low back pain during the early days of a quite short pregnancy, ending in miscarriage, can result in loss of tone, strength and control of these front muscles. But have a go!

The success rate in my classes has been high, especially with younger women (say, up to 40 years). The degree of success may depend on how young or old you are at pregnancy-time.

Chapter 7

THE GYM ROUTINE

*T*he first thing you have to do is find a gymnasium in which to do your gym routine. You may already know of one, but there could be several in your vicinity and each will differ slightly from the others. So which do you choose? The standard equipment should be very similar, but the ambience and considerations such as car parking and crèche facilities and, of course, cost will vary considerably according to who owns the gym and where it is situated. So, too, will the availability of a qualified instructor, although with this book that is not an essential requirement. The cheapest gym will probably be one run by your town, city or county council or corporation. Telephone them and they will advise you of their amenity centres and give you the appropriate telephone numbers so you can make direct enquiries. Look in Yellow Pages under 'Health Clubs and Centres', 'Leisure Centres' or 'Sports Clubs'. Ask at your sports shop or enquire at your public library. Privately run centres and clubs will be much more expensive than council ones.

If there is an instructor available at the multi-gym, make sure that he or she is qualified to teach people how to use the equipment. Make sure you emphasise that you are there to body shape only, not to body build. The equipment you use and the way you use it is specifically different for bodyshaping than for body-building. If you have any female problems, or are menstruating, you may prefer to be instructed by a qualified woman rather than a man, so that you can talk without reserve and share a mutual understanding of being a woman.

What do you wear? Anything that enables you to move your limbs without restriction, from a glamorous leotard and tights to your tatty old gardening track suit, from a pair of shorts and tee shirt to tights with the feet chopped off, your daughter's school knickers and a vest top! It doesn't matter providing the material will give and stretch as you also stretch. If you wear tights with stirrups, release these from beneath your feet or they will restrict your leg movements. You *must*, however, wear track shoes or plimsolls to protect your feet and toes while working at the equipment. They will also safeguard you from the possibility of catching athlete's foot. If you think you will want to shower afterwards, take a towel, soap and shower cap. There should, for a small further charge, be locker facilities where you can leave your clothes, shopping and purse. There may also be a crèche, but make sure that it is available at the time you want to be there or you could roll up, mid-afternoon, complete with your little one and find it's only open in the mornings!

If you are apprehensive of using a multi-gym for the first time, ask if there are group classes or go with a friend until you feel more confident. Many centres have separate gyms, one for ladies only and the other – probably the larger and better equipped – for both men and women. A multi-gym is no longer a man's world! Everyone has to start at some time, including the men that you may see straining away with sweat pouring off them. So go for it! There are sure to be certain times of day when the gym is quieter or even empty, when you can go along and study and work through this routine undisturbed. Your advantage is that you don't need an instructor if you have this book, because here you have well-explained and qualified instruction: if you work through the programme slowly and carefully to begin with and at all times observe the safety rules and the Do's and Don'ts, you will achieve the results you desire.

Remember that this form of exercise and training must remain strictly individual and non-competitive at all times. By all means ask which piece of equipment is the Latissimus Station or the Hip Flexor (you shouldn't have much trouble locating the Bicycle Machine or the Rowing Machine!) if you want to double-check. But it is *these* exercises and *this* routine which has been designed for *your* purposes and not what anyone else in the gym may kindly suggest to you.

Just take out *Bodyshaping* and start!

Before you start

You can do the entire gym routine, or selected exercises, safely three times a week only, leaving at least one day in between. The maximum time you spend in the gym, including warm-up sequence, rests and relaxation will be about three-quarters to one hour.

Any muscle that is regularly worked must tone up, lose fat and therefore change shape.

Be aware of the difference between bodyshaping and body-building.

To Bodyshape: regulate the weights just enough to provide sufficient resistance and exercise fairly fast. Gradually increase the resistance (but not too much) so that it is always there, or work faster. This will tone and reduce.

To Body-build: regulate the weights to provide maximum resistance. Your muscles will have to work more slowly and much harder. This will tone and develop them.

Safety first

Remember: to make sure *first* that:

● You have the correct weight (under rather than over) and the safety-pin is homed correctly. With the exception of the first weight, which will always move up and down, all subsequent weights need to have the safety-pin fixed into the slot beneath them. At whatever level of weight you fix the pin, all weights above it will move up and down, en bloc, as you control the equipment to which they are attached. On most makes of equipment, the safety-pin slips into the space provided. You then give it a sideways twist which secures it. Check it is secure and you are ready to begin.

● The sloping benches are fixed securely.

When you are using the multi-gym equipment you are working your body against the resistance of weights and equipment. You must always be in control of them. They must NEVER get the better of you (this is how injury and accidents occur). You are responsible for not overdoing it. Control the speed of the weights as they return; this exercises the same muscles. *Breathe out on effort* – you will find the work easier because this sets a rhythm. Be slightly breathless as this proves you are exercising your heart and lungs, and your aerobic performance will improve.

Sets and repetitions

Gradually increase the number of repetitions within a set, e.g. 3x5, 3x7, 3x9, etc. Rest between each set at the chosen equipment, then go on to the next piece, i.e. complete work at one station and don't return to it.

Isometrics

You can exercise your muscles isometrically using gym equipment. At the level where you feel the appropriate muscles working their hardest, hold for *7 seconds only*, *once a day only*.

Do's and don'ts

1. DO exercise regularly, if you want results.

2. DO rest between sets.

3. DO stop and rest in a vertical position should you feel dizzy.

4. DO wear shoes in the gymnasium (as opposed to barefoot for the warm-up sequence). Your feet need protection against the equipment, and against catching athlete's foot.

5. DO exercise your abdominal muscles *last*.

6. NEVER work through pain. Pain is telling you that something is wrong and that you should attend to it. See your GP.

7. NEVER exercise in the gym if you are pregnant, trying to become pregnant or have just had your baby. If you have a history of heart irregularities or medical or structural problems, see your GP.

8. NEVER attempt inverted positions if you have high blood pressure (you will have seen your GP first for high blood pressure).

9. NEVER assist another person to use equipment. Weighted equipment must be controlled only by the person primarily responsible and for whose benefit it is being used.

10. DON'T let your young daughter exercise in a multi-gym if she is *pre-puberty:* her body is growing towards an important phase of development. Her bones are still forming and hardening and at the same time her muscles which move them are becoming very powerful. Her sacrum and coccyx bones at the base of her spine are

finally fusing together. Pre-puberty, this form of exercise could affect her bone structure and development adversely, permanently.

11. DON'T eat a big meal beforehand. Stick to 'light and small, or not at all'.

12. NEVER allow young children into a gymnasium, even if you or other adults are there as well. Young children may be tempted to play on the equipment, or stand close to it while it is being used, and they could be seriously injured. You cannot work effectively yourself *and* keep an eye on them. Accidents happen when your back is turned for that fleeting moment, and the responsibility is yours. The gymnasium should have a rule about children not entering the gym. Make sure *you* keep it.

The Routine

ALWAYS DO THE BREATHING EXERCISE AND WARM-UP SEQUENCE FIRST.

1. Breathing exercise

Breathe deeply, slowly, 3 or 4 times.

2. Warm-up sequence

3. Equipment

Points to remember:

Exercise from toe to top, abdomen exercises 11 & 12 *always last*

1. **Stretch rib-cage** 'passively' (at Latissimus Station): Kneel close to equipment, keep bottom on heels throughout. Let the weights do the work but you must have control.

2. **Ankles, calves** (at Leg Press): Legs straight all the time, toes only on pad. Bend and straighten ankles.

3. **Thighs** – inside outside (at Ankle Strap): Fit foot into strap, hold on to machine. Pull leg *out* to side to exercise *out*side thigh; keeping same foot in strap, turn around and pull leg *across* body and up, to exercise *in*side thigh.

4. **Thighs** – front (Quadriceps muscles) (at Leg back (Hamstring muscles) Conditioner): To exercise front of thigh: sit, feet under lower pads, raise legs. To exercise back of thigh: lie on tummy, feet under upper pads, bend knees.

5. **Legs overall** (at Bicycle Machine).

6. **Body overall** (at Rowing Machine): Don't continue for too long at these two machines if you find them easy, because you still have more work to do!

7. **Chest** (at Chest Conditioner): Lie on back, shoulders under bar, hands close, push up.

8. **Back of upper arm** (Triceps muscle) against chair or bench: a) start with bent elbows
   b) straighten arms
   Take weight of body by having feet on ground. Keep body clear of bench. Push on hands to straighten arms.

9. **Shoulders** (at Press Station):
   Sit on stool, tuck feet around stool legs, shoulders directly under bar, push up.

10. **Shoulders, Upper back, Upper chest** (at Latissimus Station):
    As No. 1; pull bar down behind head, then in front of head. This time, *you* do the work.

11. **Abdomen** (at Abdominal Conditioner):
    Start with low bench. Raise straight legs. If 'hollow back' is uncomfortable, leave out this equipment.

12. **Abdomen** (at Hip Flexor):
    Keep low back pressed into padding.

Breathe *in* before effort and *out* on effort throughout the routine.

4. Relax

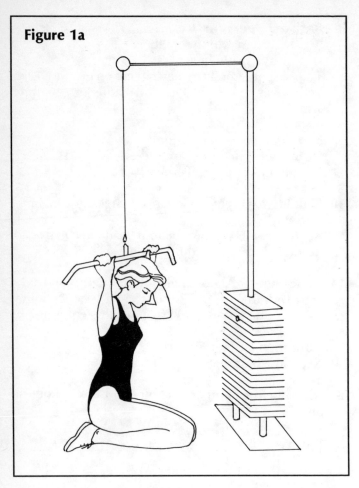

Figure 1a

1   Stretch rib-cage – *at Latissimus Station*
1x7

Secure the pin under the required number of weights. Three weights is average for a woman.

SP   Kneel quite close to the equipment, sitting back on your heels, directly under the bar. Keep your bottom on your heels throughout the exercise. Pull the bar down

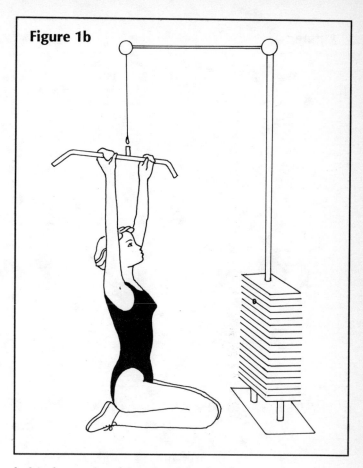

Figure 1b

behind your head, to shoulder level.

Allow the bar to rise up until your arms are straight and your rib-cage feels comfortably 'stretched'. Then pull the bar down to SP again. Repeat 7 times. Relax.

This is one set of 7 repetitions (1x7).

This is the only 'passive' exercise in the routine, in that you are allowing an external influence, in this case the weights, to do the work. But you must still have control of what is happening.

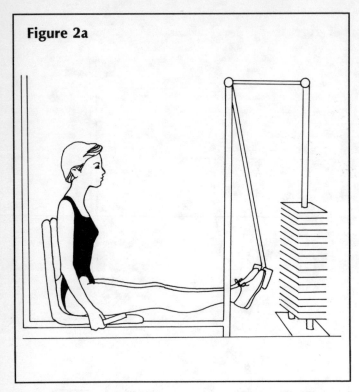

Figure 2a

2 Ankles, calves – *at Leg Press Station*
3x5

Secure the pin under the required number of weights.

SP Sit in the chair, hold the hand grips (the chair can be adjusted to accommodate your individual leg length). Straight legs, toes only on the foot pad.

Point your feet, pushing the foot pad away from you, then relax them back to SP. Keep your knees straight throughout the exercise. 5 times. Relax.

This exercises all the joints in your feet and ankles, and the muscles that work these joints. You should feel the work in your calves in particular.

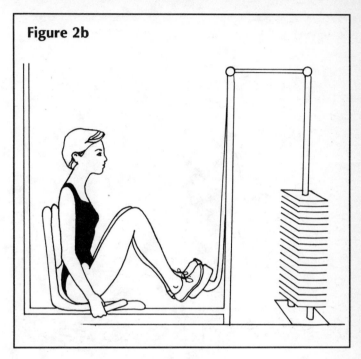

Figure 2b

Another way to use this station: 3x5

SP   Sit in the chair as before but with your knees bent up and the whole of your feet on the foot pad.

Straighten your knees, relax to SP. 5 times. Relax.

You will now feel the muscles working at the front of your thighs because it is this large group of muscles that is responsible for straightening your knees.

This exercises in particular your knee joints and thighs. You may decide *not* to include this second movement in your gym routine because it is quite strong. Most women exercise their knees quite enough during each day, by dint of their daily routine, not to require it. It is intended more for men who wish to build up their thigh muscles. There are other movements in the routine which adequately attend to your knees and thighs e.g. 3, 4, 5.

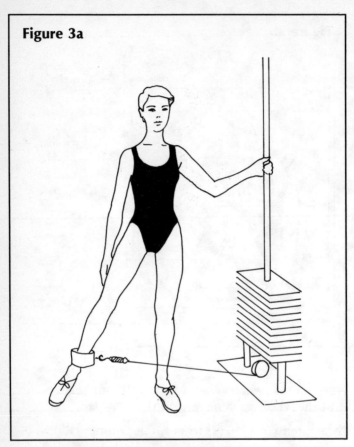

Figure 3a

3   Thighs – inside/outside
at Ankle Strap Station   3x3

This is an excellent exercise for shaping and reducing those bulgy inner and outer thighs, but it's hard work!

Secure the pin under the required number of weights.

SP   With L side to the equipment, stand on your L leg and slip your R foot into the ankle strap. Hold on to the equipment to keep your balance and prevent your body

Figure 3b

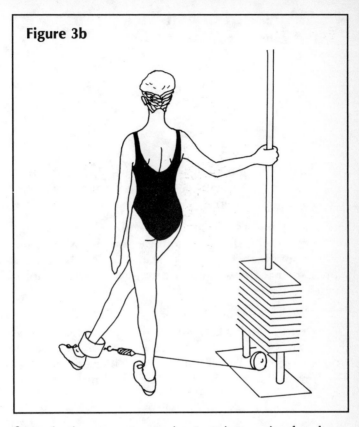

from tipping as you exercise (causing strain elsewhere, especially at low back and abdomen).

Move your R straight leg sideways away from the equipment, out and up. 3 times. This exercises your outside thigh.

Still balancing on your L leg, turn around so that your R side is next to the equipment and with your R foot still in the ankle strap. Pull your R straight leg in front and across your balancing leg, away from the equipment, across and up. 3 times. This exercises your inside thigh.

This is one set of 3 repetitions (1x3).

4   Thighs – front and back
at Leg Conditioner   3x3

Secure the pin under the required number of weights.

Front thighs

SP   Sit on the end of the bench with your knees bent over the end and your feet tucked under the lower footpads. Support your body on straight arms.

Breathe in, and as you breathe out straighten your legs. This will raise the footpads and weights. You should feel your front thigh muscles working. Slowly bend your knees so that the weights gently lower, without noise. Repeat 3 times. Relax.
This is 1 set of 3 repetitions (1x3)

To extend Lean back in your sitting position and move your hands back on the bench to support your body. Repeat exercise. You should feel the effect on your front thigh muscles and your low abdominal muscles.

Back thighs

SP   Lie on your tummy and tuck your heels under the upper footpads.

Breathe in, and as you breathe out bend your knees, raising the footpads and weights. When you feel the effect to maximum on your back thigh muscles gently allow the weights to lower to SP. Repeat 3 times. Relax.

This is 1 set of 3 repetitions (1x3).

Both these exercises can be held isometrically at the point of greatest effort on the working muscles.

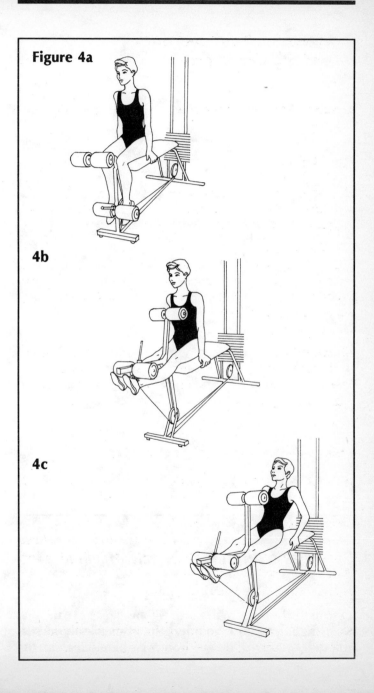

Figure 4a

4b

4c

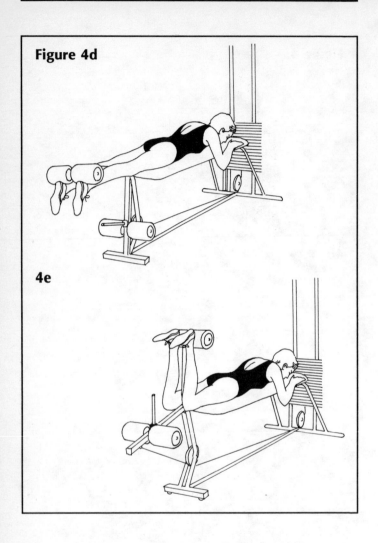

Figure 4d

4e

5   Legs overall – *at Bicycle Machine*

For a comfortable length of time.

One of the bicycles in the gym will perhaps have the seat at the right height for your length of legs. If not, the seat will adjust up or down. You will find dials on the

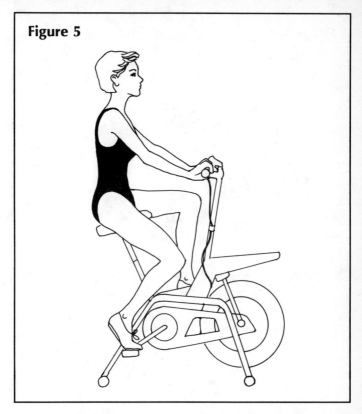

Figure 5

handlebars which will show you the mileage and speed at which you are cycling, and a dial which you can adjust to produce the resistance against which you work. If you are not able to make the adjustments yourself ask one of the staff, or another gym-user, to help you.

Now ride your bike! And cycle until your leg and hip muscles feel well worked. Stop for a rest every now and then. If your muscles start to feel shaky, because you are unused to this exercise or you are beginning to overdo it – stop at once and rest and do no more. Nature is telling you that you've done enough. Practice will increase your ability – this is what it's all about. Never distress yourself. Exercise should be a pleasure.

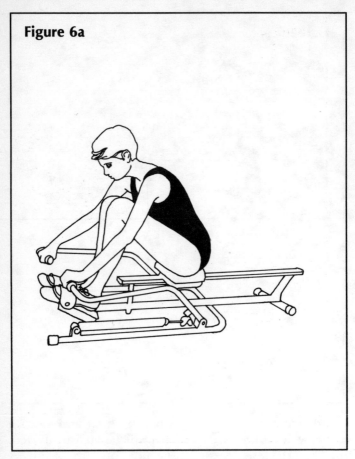

Figure 6a

6 Body overall – *at Rowing Machine*

For a comfortable length of time.

Again, if necessary readjust the seat so that it is the right distance away from the foot pads for your own leg length. You will find a knob at about hand level, on each side, which you can adjust to increase or decrease the resistance at which you 'row'. Adjust this pressure so that it is equal on both sides to make sure that your body works in a straight line. Slip your feet under the straps

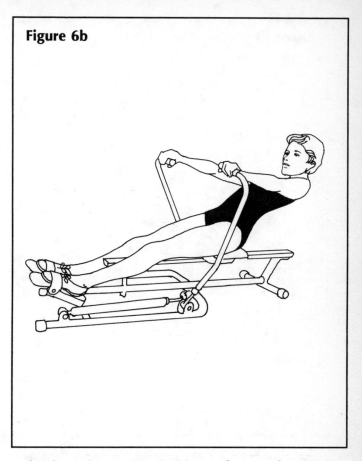

Figure 6b

and tighten the straps to hold your feet comfortably but firmly.

Breathe *in* on least effort, as your body moves forward towards your feet, and *out* as you exert yourself pulling backwards. It may take a while to acquire this habit but the rowing is easier, more effective and you will sustain it for longer.

Now row your boat! Row until you begin to tire. Rest. Start again. Rest. As with the bicycle machine, don't overdo it.

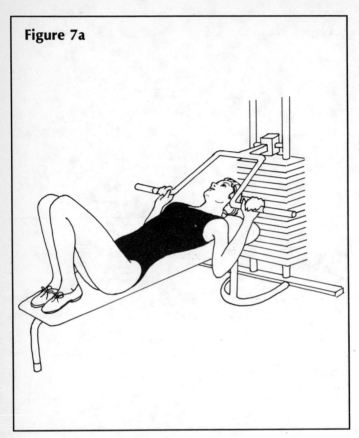

Figure 7a

7 **Chest –** *at Chest Conditioner* 3x3

Exercise at this station if you want to increase and tone up your chest muscles. It may increase your bust measurement but will not increase your actual breast size because they consist of fatty tissues, not muscles. Therefore you may not want to use this station.

Secure the pin under the required number of weights.

SP Lie on the bench, on your back, with your shoulders directly under the bar. Bend your knees with your feet on the end of the bench, to take any undue strain off your

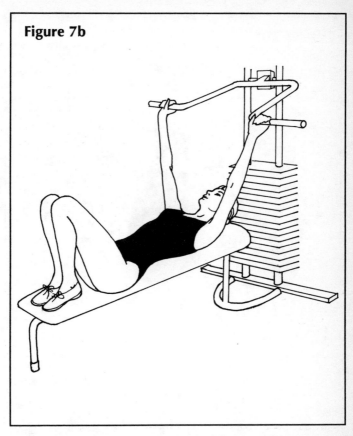

Figure 7b

abdominal muscles and low back. Grasp the bar with your hands at a point above your shoulders.

Breathe in. As you breathe out, push bar up, straightening your arms. Relax to SP as you breathe in. Repeat 3 times. Relax.

This forms 1 set of 3 repetitions (1x3).

If you want to tone up (and possibly develop) your shoulder muscles (deltoid muscle) place your hands wider apart on the bar before exercising. This uses your shoulders more.

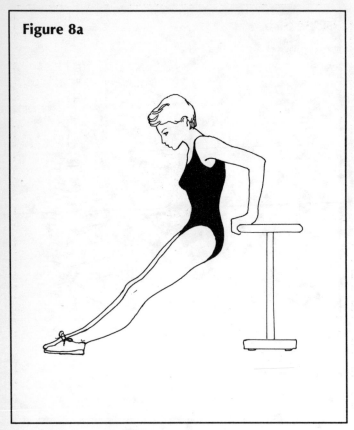

Figure 8a

8   Back of upper arm
against chair or bench   3x5

The back of the upper arm is an area that often becomes flabby and toneless as women grow older. This exercise is excellent for toning up this triceps muscle.

Make sure the bench or chair against which you are working will not slip.

SP   Sit on the bench with your hands holding the edge of the seat, legs straight. Lower your body off the bench by sliding your straight legs forwards and bending your

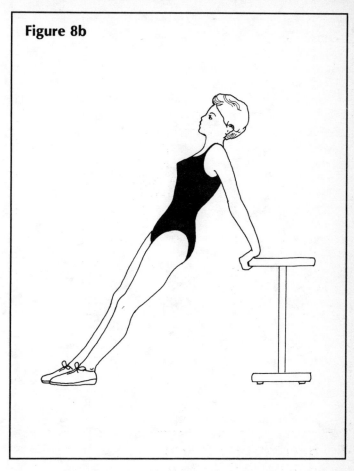

Figure 8b

elbows, keeping your bottom clear of the floor, as in the diagram. Push on your hands to straighten your arms but keep your feet in the same place. Your entire body should be in a straight line from feet to shoulders. Return to SP by bending your elbows. Remember to breathe out on effort and in as your body relaxes back to SP. Keep your legs straight throughout this exercise. Five times. Relax

This forms 1 set of 5 repetitions.

To extend Hold the 5th time isometrically.

Figure 9a

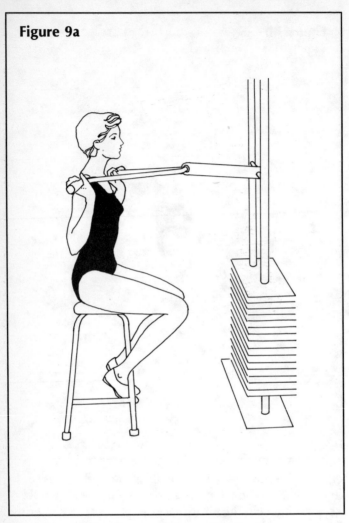

9 Shoulders – *at Press Station* 3x5

Secure the pin under the required number of weights.

SP Place a stool before the equipment and sit on it, with your shoulders directly below the bar. Tuck your feet around the stool legs for stability. Grasp bar.

Figure 9b

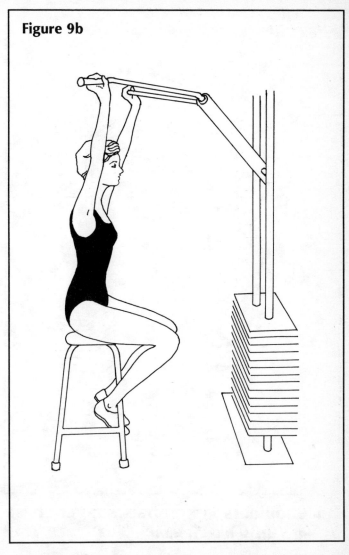

Breathe in. As you breathe out, push the bar up to straighten your arms. Relax to SP as you breathe in. Three times. Relax.

This forms 1 set of 3 repetitions (1x3).

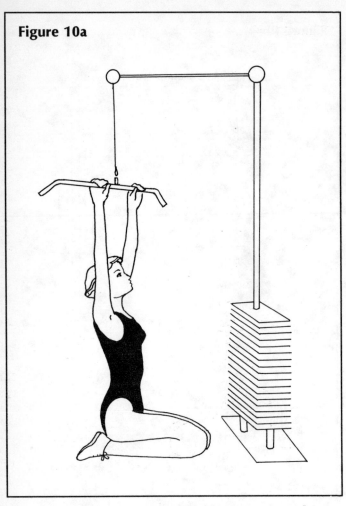

Figure 10a

10 Shoulders, upper back, upper chest
at Latissimus Station   3x3

Secure the pin at the required number of weights.

SP   Kneel quite close to the equipment, sitting back on your heels, directly under the bar. Grasp the bar with both hands, straight arms.

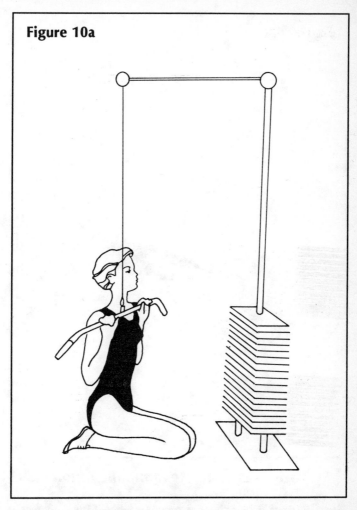

Figure 10a

Breathe in. Breathe out as you pull the bar down behind your head. Breathe in as you let the bar rise. Breathe out as you pull the bar down in front of your head. Breathe in as you let the bar rise again. Three times. Relax.
This forms 1 set of 3 repetitions (1x3).

Don't clonk yourself on the head as you do this exercise!

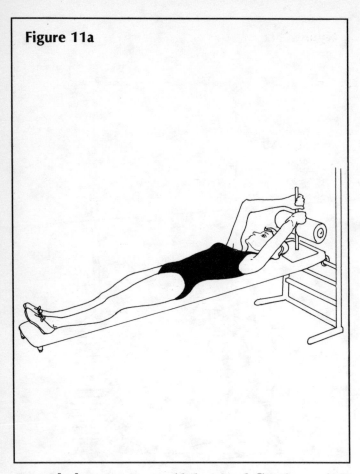

Figure 11a

11 Abdomen – *at Abdominal Station* 3x3

Start with the bench at a gentle slope. Make sure it is safely hooked into position.

SP Lie on your back on the bench with your head towards the top end, clasp the handles firmly.

Raise straight legs until you feel the pull on your working abdominal muscles. Relax to SP. Three times. Relax. This forms 1 set of 3 repetitions (1x3)

Figure 11b

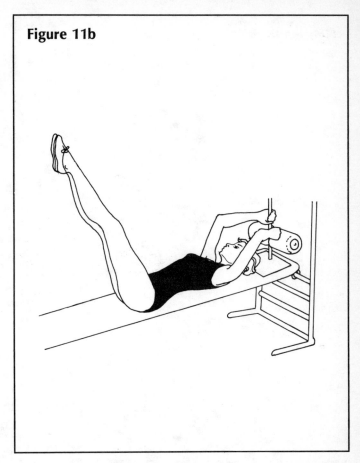

This is a very powerful abdominal exercise. Because some of your abdominal muscles originate on your low spine you may experience a degree of discomfort in your 'hollow back' area. In this case do not use this piece of equipment.

To extend The last time that you raise your legs hold the position isometrically.
Also to extend: Fix the bench securely at a steeper slope. Your abdominal muscles will work more strongly in order to raise your legs.

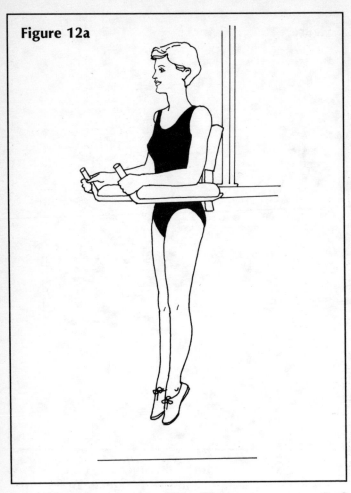

Figure 12a

12 Abdomen – *at Hip Flexor* 3x3

SP Climb up to the equipment with, perhaps, the use of a stool. Place your arms along the length of the arm rests for support. Grasp the handles and 'hang' from the equipment.

Keep your low back pressed into the padding throughout the exercise.

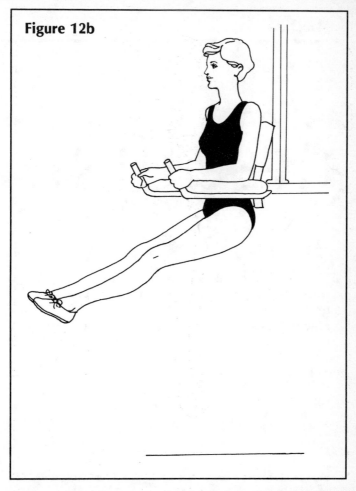

Figure 12b

Raise straight legs into the air. Relax to SP. Repeat 3 times. Relax.

This forms 1 set of 3 repetitions (1x3).

NOW LIE FLAT ON THE FLOOR AND RELAX UNTIL YOU ARE AWARE THAT YOUR BREATHING AND HEART BEAT HAVE QUIETENED AFTER YOUR EXERCISING.

Chapter 8

A-Z of
TIPS & HINTS

*T*his is a selective list of hints, tips and tried-and-tested natural remedies for minor but irritating problems. Of course, you must always refer to your doctor should a problem persist, but some of the 'old wives' remedies' can be just as effective as any modern and expensive techno-treatment. You will probably be able to add your own favourite remedies to the list.

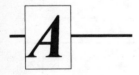

Aching or sore feet

In a washing up bowl, add 15 ml/1 tablespoon of sea salt and 5 ml/1 teaspoonful of bicarbonate of soda to 2 litres/ 4 pints of hot water. Soak your feet and rest for 15 minutes.

Acid stomach

This is often caused by too much protein or by not
chewing your food enough. Goat's milk yoghurt may
help. Ensure that your teeth and/or dentures are in
working order, enabling you to chew properly.

Antiseptics

Natural antiseptics include your own saliva! Lick the
wound (if you can reach it) like animals do. You have a
natural healing element transferred via your tongue.
Other 100 per cent sterile products include honey,
onion, garlic. Including these in your diet will help
healing processes. (Should you store these in containers
with metal lids they begin to lose their antiseptic quality
as soon as they come into contact with metal.)

Arthritis

This can affect the hands and fingers in particular. Your
hands are probably the most brilliant machine ever
created. Your natural functions from birth mostly curl
them inwards: clutching your rattle, gripping bicycle
handlebars, pushing a pram, grasping door handles,
writing with pen and pencil, knitting, carrying baskets,
etc. Tension also makes you curl them inwards. In later
life it can be difficult to stretch them out at all. Many
people sleep with closed fists, from habit. Train yourself
to go to sleep with your hands unclenched. Place your
open hands under your tummy, chest or pillow so that
the weight of these keeps them open, until it becomes a
habit to prepare for sleep this way. When you lie on the
floor, kneel down to use a dustpan and brush or bend
down to pick something up, train yourself to stand up
again by balancing in a crouching position and then

pushing off with straight, splayed fingers. Use this method all the time; it counteracts that inward, flexing movement.

Attitude of mind

Thought is all-powerful and it is possible to cultivate a mental attitude of, say, cheerfulness, happiness, positiveness or success which can only be beneficial to your living and also the success of a slimming and exercising programme. It's truly said 'It's all in the mind'.

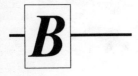

Back

The first sign of spring and the gardeners get busy. So do the osteopaths and masseuses! If you dig and weed and hoe all day, whether it's slight bending over or down on your knees, you may ache the next day. But before then you may have the problem of actually straightening yourself up! When the sun comes out and the climate is milder we lose all sense of moderation. Here are two ways to ease your overworked back.

Exercise one

SP   Stand straight, feet together, hands placed lightly on the front of your thighs.

Starting with your *head*, slowly drop your head and gently let your spine curl forwards as far down as you can comfortably go. Keep your neck relaxed throughout, and your hands in contact with your legs as you drop downwards to help you to maintain your balance. If you reach the point where it is uncomfortable to go any further, this is the place where most stress has concentrated during your day-long activity. If you know that usually you can drop further forward than this, see if by dint of relaxing you can pass through this point and continue down. When you have reached as low as you can go, without force, slowly and gently straighten up passing through the same trouble spot until you are straight again, making sure your neck is the last bit of your spine to straighten. Be aware of each vertebral joint flexing and extending, one by one, as you curve down and curve up. Always start and end with your neck. (If you keep your neck straight this tension will reflect itself throughout your spine and there will be no benefit.) Bend and straighten like this, gently, 3 times.

This is for immediate relief during the day's gardening and also at the end of the day's session. It gently exercises the muscles and joints that have become stressed through unaccustomed, prolonged and maybe over-enthusiastic use. If you suffer from back tension at any time this is an excellent exercise to bring relief.

If you have any back *problems* you should be seeing a professional for medical help.

Exercise two

This exercise is more dramatic, for otherwise healthy backs. The idea is to take out the strain with a sudden 'shock' movement.

SP Stand with feet apart and bend your knees keeping your feet flat on the floor; bend your body forwards and rest your elbows on top of your knees, hands dangling towards the floor. This should be quite a stable position.

Suddenly release your elbows off your knees so that your body drops forwards. The sudden movement can often release that ache at low spine level. Repeat 3 times in all.

Other ways to help yourself:

Do exercise 23 in the warm-up sequence (see page 113). Soak in a hot bath. This helps to take the tension out of your muscles. Do a few gentle spine exercises afterwards.

Balance

Catch phrases don't arise without reason. 'The balance of nature'. 'A balanced way of living'. 'A proper balance'. 'Maintaining your balance'. 'Weighed in the balance (and found wanting?)' 'Do the scales balance?'

If you live with the emphasis, or bias, directed too much in one way or another, perhaps physically, mentally or emotionally, the stress of that imbalance is detrimental to you. Nature always balances for us but we give her a hard time sometimes! This book is all about balance.

An emotional imbalance can be remedied by creative pursuits. Truly creative people are rarely emotionally imbalanced. Too much mental bias in your life can be assisted by physical activities.

Bathing

A warm or hot bath is more relaxing than showering but probably less refreshing. A shower after exercise may remove sweat more effectively but will stimulate you. If you are ill or very tired you may find that a bath will take away energy rather than restore it and you should perhaps avoid bathing at these times. A warm bath will also relax your muscles before certain kinds of exercise, for example before practising yoga which is in itself teaching you to relax.

Bending and stretching

Bending and stretching exercises your joints within the direction that they are designed to move. They only move because your muscles operate them, so all bending and stretching movements keep you flexible and active, can help or delay arthritis and help to prevent ageing. If you play golf or go bowling or walk you are not bending and stretching all over – and it is the all over that is so beneficial and effective. The warm-up sequence couldn't be better for you. Domestically, make sure that you really bend down to that lowest shelf in the cupboard, bend your knees and hips (don't stick out your bottom with half straight legs! Apart from being ungainly it's a strain on your low back). Kneel to clean the floor. Stretch up on tip-toe to that top shelf and have your shelves sufficiently high to make you do so. But, of course, don't strain yourself or that is going to the other extreme and is dangerous.

Stretch when you get up in the morning (or while you are in bed), stretch after a relaxing bath, stretch after exercise and after a relaxing snooze. It's like a physical all-over yawn. Bending and stretching is also very beneficial for constipation sufferers. (See warm-up sequence exercise 1.)

Bloatedness

This feels very uncomfortable and when severe you become enlarged and 'bloated' at waist and abdomen so that it may be difficult even to fasten up your skirt at the waistband. Keep off solid food for 24 hours, sipping water only in small quantities. Rest. When you eat make sure it is easily digested food like white bread or scrambled egg. Curl into a small shape and slowly uncurl. If you tend to bloatedness, due to leaving it too long between meals, then eat smaller meals more frequently. (See *Fluid retention* also).

Blowing your nose

If you are stuffed up in your nostrils or sinuses or generally in your eustachian tubes, don't blow your nose with any force. The passages in your nose, mouth and ears are interconnected and violent nose-blowing of both nostrils at the same time builds up pressure because you have closed off both airways at the same time. It can cause your ears to 'pop' and continued violent blowing of both nostrils at the same time might even damage your inner ear drums. When using your hanky or tissue, close one nostril and blow down the other one, then reverse the procedure. This prevents the pressure from building up because as you blow you still have a free air passage via the other nostril.

Natural remedies to help you clear blocked-up nasal and sinus systems are: breathing in the scent of myrrh, frankincense, eucalyptus or roses. You may have a local health store, homeopathic chemist or herbal therapist who can provide you with these. Eucalyptus kernels in your room or rose petals in a pot pourri will retain their fragrance for a long time. Douche your nasal passages occasionally with salt and bicarbonate of soda (600 ml/1 pint warm water to 5 ml/1 teaspoon salt and a large pinch of bicarbonate of soda).

Breathing

This is a natural and involuntary function of your existence. Tension tightens your respiratory system. Smoking clogs up your lungs and prevents vital nutritious oxygen from passing into your blood stream. So does pollution in the atmosphere. The best possible breathing pattern helps you to resist the damage of these poisons and also to recover from colds, viruses and illnesses should they occur. Keeping your rib-cage and abdominal muscles in good trim will promote good breathing patterns.

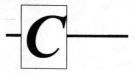

Carrying

Hold articles close to your body so that their centre of gravity and yours combine a little and you become more like one and less like two. This takes strain off your arms and saves your back, and of course means less strain on your abdominal muscles. This is particularly applicable when you carry small children. Don't carry anything that is too heavy or too large and awkward without help. Distribute heavy articles, like shopping, equally in each hand.

Cats and dogs

Your domestic cat lives by instinct in a way that we should watch and learn from. It tends to eat only when it is hungry and stops eating when it's had enough. Also, if it feels unwell it will stop eating to allow its system to recover. *We* call this 'going off our food' but often we don't allow our instincts to take over and we still continue to eat. A cat can also be quite particular about what it eats. Dogs aren't always like this, but both stretch after sleep or a rest period, to limber-in before more energetic activity. This is what we have to do with the warm-up sequence before the gym routine! Your domestic pet stretches the front half of the body followed by each hind leg, one after the other. Children stretch a lot, but adults have mostly lost the art. It's worth re-educating yourself this way and the more relaxed you are the more instinctive it will become (see *Bending and stretching*).

Cellulite

If your thighs look like cottage cheese you have not necessarily left it too late but don't leave it any longer! Cellulite is an updated name for congealed fat! You find these areas mostly on your thighs and they are made up of too many poorly distributed fat cells. A slimming diet will start to take away the fat and the right exercise will start to tone you up in the right places. You are more likely to have cellulite if you have a slow metabolism and are overweight. Massage at these areas helps to improve the circulation and remove unwanted tissues.

Chesty catarrh

If you don't mind garlic and its anti-social tendencies, here is a recipe that loosens chesty catarrh and phlegm.

Crush half a clove of garlic and half a medium-sized onion in a garlic crusher. Place this in a glass bowl, or jam jar, and cover with *runny* honey. Leave it for six hours. If necessary top up with honey after the first hour as the honey drains through the garlic and onion and they need to be covered. Drain off the liquid, through muslin or a plastic sieve. Sip a teaspoonful (5ml) every four hours. You should cough up phlegm within minutes.

Store the garlic mixture in the fridge indefinitely, in a plastic or glass bowl, covered, but not using a metal lid. The above mixture is free from micro-organisms but if it touches metal (other than pre-1920 silver) it will begin to spoil.

Cold weather

The cold is bracing only if you brace yourself to it. If you shrink from it your system shrinks too and does not build up a resistance to cope, especially in your respiratory system. This is how colds and coughs can start. Wear warm but loose clothing to allow an airflow around your body. Graduate the temperature when you return indoors. Many houses and offices have central heating turned up so high that our bodies can't adjust between outdoors and indoors without succumbing to colds and dry throats. There should always be a jug of water in every centrally-heated room to moisten the atmosphere and prevent *us* from drying out, and a window open to allow the air to circulate. It is always healthier indoors to keep the temperature lower and wear an extra loose-fitting sweater or a thermal under-garment.

Perhaps you huddle into your clothes or find it difficult to face the elements because you lack self-confidence or feel insecure. If you can learn to enjoy the elements, you can overcome many other difficulties.

Constipation

Prolonged constipation is a slow poisoning of the entire system because you are not getting rid of waste matter. You know what happens to your drains if you don't keep them clear! If you are prone to constipation, you can tackle it in the following way until it no longer occurs. Keep off eggs because the yolks are binding, and so is hard cheese. Drink three glasses of water daily. Eat sufficient fibre. Use herbal laxatives if necessary in preference to non-herbal ones because they are gentler and more natural to your body. Cauliflower florets and lettuce leaves are a natural laxative. Curling up positions will put pressure on your abdomen to act as a self-massage. If you use your hands on your abdomen in an attempt to relieve constipation only use flat pressure and not circular movements because you cannot tell which point your 'blockage' has reached in its journey along your intestines. Never let anyone other than a qualified practitioner massage your abdomen. Massage to relieve constipation is a highly technical treatment.

Watch the way animals squat as they relieve their

bowels. If you keep a footstool, about 20 cm/8 in high, in your bathroom and rest your feet on this when you are sitting down on the lavatory you can effect this squatting position and make the daily function easier.

Because what happens at one end of the system affects the other end, constipation can give you headaches or migraine. Constipation can be caused by tension.

If you suffer from prolonged constipation, see your doctor.

Cracks on finger tips

These can be very painful and take a long time to heal. They can be caused by not wearing rubber or protective gloves for wet, dry or dirty work; by touching hot things like hot pans, hot toast, jacket potatoes straight from the oven or newly-boiled eggs from the pan. Use natural washing-up liquids and soap powders rather than detergent-based ones. Go to your homoeopathic chemist for silicea-graphite pillules. Cut down on your egg intake. Take vitamin B for a while.

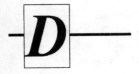

Diarrhoea

Including an egg or hard cheese into your diet may help because they have a binding effect. Or, for 24-48 hours, don't eat solid foods to give your system a rest and a chance to balance. Don't forget you are losing fluid, so never cut down on drinking.

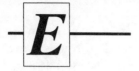

Early-in-the-day foods

Proteins require greater digesting so eat them early in the day, so that you have the day ahead not only for the digesting process but for reaping the benefits they provide. Cheese particularly should be eaten earlier rather than later.

Enjoyment

Enjoyment brings relaxation of the mind and a sense of well-being. Many people think that to be happy, or enjoy their living, is something that is somehow not permitted. Why not?! A lot of it is learning how to be oneself and how to stop apologising, either to others or to one's self, for one's existence.

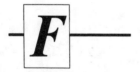

Fanaticism

Fanaticism is excess in one direction or another and is therefore imbalance and not healthy. Excess of anything is contrary to nature and can actually increase ill-health. Our immune system balances itself all the time that we treat our system with reasonable respect and moderation, as in our eating and exercising. Scientific studies have confirmed that really intensive exercise, for example, can suppress the immune system.

Fibre

Fibre, or roughage, is necessary in your diet to provide bulk for the passage of your food through your alimentary canal. Too much fibre can constipate you, and can also cause weight gain. Too little fibre can also cause constipation as your system cannot work properly without it. Once again we are talking about getting the balance right for the person that you are. There are plenty of books on the market that will tell you all about fibre, giving well-tried and recommended recipes.

Flatulence

This is very unpleasant and causes you to burp and pass wind and have an enlarged abdomen and a sensitive stomach that is sometimes tender to touch. Perhaps you have eaten too much raw salad or vegetables? Try sipping a cup of yarrow tea. Yarrow herbs, from your health store, are inexpensive. Goat's milk yoghurt is good for flatulence and should be available at your health store.

Here is a good exercise to help to relieve flatulence.

SP Lie on your back on the floor.

Breathe deeply through your nose. Hold your breath in as you curl your knees up to your chest and clasp your hands round them to keep your bent legs pulled in close to your body. When you feel your face begin to flush, release your legs, let your breath out noisily through your mouth and relax to SP. Repeat 3 times. With any luck the pressure of your legs against your abdomen and stomach area, which are extended because you are holding your breath in, will force any gassiness out of your body as you release the pressure and relax.

Fluid retention

Too much bread, or other high sodium content food, may be the cause of this problem. If you cut down on bread and similar carbohydrates and follow a slimming diet and all-over exercise programme you may well discover that your clothes begin to be loose on you and rings that have been apparently too small for a long time slip easily on to your fingers again (see also *Bloatedness*).

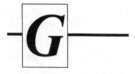

Gardening

For those of you who love to garden, this can be one of the best therapies to unwind mentally, relax and therefore heal.

Gut feeling

The importance of your abdominal area has already been stressed. Your digestive system (along with your respiratory system) works by involuntary process. Because digestion is supremely important, necessary for maintaining life, nature doesn't let you attend to it yourself on a voluntary basis! It is also the area of your body where really well-toned and strong muscles are required, to protect your internal organs and to protect and expand whilst your baby is developing inside you. Your abdominal muscles work strongly when you cough, sneeze, vomit, urinate, defaecate and during childbirth.

This area would seem to have a more subtle importance. Why do we say 'I have a gut feeling' or 'it took a lot of guts'?

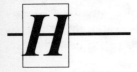

Hair

Is your hair your crowning glory? A good hairdresser will advise you best on the kind of shampoo you should be using to give you healthy, well-conditioned and shiny hair. If you are unwell, your hair is one of the first areas to reflect your state of health. A dry scalp will produce dry, lack-lustre hair. When you wash your hair, massage your scalp thoroughly with your finger tips. Include lightly boiled cabbage and carrots into your diet. A drop of corn oil with your food helps, too.

Headaches

If you have persistent headaches you must do something about it. Are you constipated? Are you consuming too much cheese, chocolate or coffee? Avoid gin, white meat, rhubarb and pork. Your diet probably needs a complete overhaul. Learn to relax, mentally and physically (perhaps by the study and practice of yoga). Have you a structural problem, or tension, in your feet or at the base of your spine? The energy in your body is constantly travelling and interacting in response to how you are, physically, mentally and emotionally. Energy manifesting itself as pain, tension or a physical problem at the base of your spine may travel up your spine to lodge in your neck, or vice versa. Your headache may be the result of stress at low spine level. (See also *Migraine*.)

Herbs to help you slim

Try fennel seed and chives. Infuse fennel seed and drink it as tea, to the strength that suits your palate. (You can buy fennel seed tea bags.) Add fresh chives to your raw foods, such as salads, into your sandwiches and into your cooking of vegetables. Both these herbs help to clean the bloodstream, permitting a better flow and proper elimination of toxins, thus speeding up your metabolism.

Hiccups

Providing that you do not laugh or giggle while you attempt this cure for hiccups, you should be able to get rid of them.

Fill a glass with warm water, to the brim, and ask a friend to stand in front of you and hold it up to your mouth. Raise your arms straight up above your head, lean forward and sip from the *far* side of the glass. You may well put your chin in the water or dribble. Sip 3 or 4 times, with quiet concentration. After the hiccups stop, lower your arms and breathe very slowly and quietly for a minute or two so that your body can return to its normal breathing pattern.

Raising your arms and leaning over the glass lifts your rib-cage up and 'fixes it' for a moment or two, while your quiet concentration helps to break the abnormal breathing pattern that often causes hiccups.

Hollow back

This uncomfortable condition seems to be a woman's complaint and can run, almost genetically, in the women in a family. It is a tightening and accentuation of the spinal curve in the lumbar region. Here are some excellent movements to assist you, as it is possible completely to get rid of it.

Exercise one

SP   Lie on your back on the floor, with your knees bent up and your feet on the floor, resting your hands over your waist.

Press that 'hollow-back' area into the floor, hold a moment, relax to SP. Repeat several times.

Exercise two

Learn to lie down, from sitting position, as follows.

SP   Sit on the floor with your knees bent up and your feet on the floor, then lean your trunk backwards until you take the weight of your body on your elbows, with your forearms on the floor.

Gradually curve your spine down to the floor, unfolding it vertebra by vertebra on to the floor until your hollow back is no longer 'hollow' but is completely in contact with the floor. As you put your head to the floor straighten your arms by your side. Pause for a moment and then very slowly let your legs relax to a straight position until you are lying quietly. Letting your legs straighten will bring back the 'hollow' because there is naturally a curve in that area but with practice it will become less pronounced. You must complete this exercise through to the end each time because you are aiming to achieve this eased back for when you are standing and sitting, not just lying.

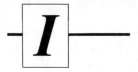

Ingrowing toenails

Working on the principle that a problem at one end of your body can cause a problem at the other end of your body, an ingrowing toenail on your big toe can cause headaches and migraine. Keeping the cuticles soft, especially at the top and side, makes it easier to check what is happening to the nail itself. You can rub in oil occasionally or use a cuticle cream from the chemist. Keep your toenails short and cut them squarely across. Make sure there is enough room in the toes of your shoes to accommodate your toes without them being squashed together. Wear stockings or tights that are *not gathered* into a top toe seam but are seamed across the top with a straight seam. If the problem is severe, consult your doctor or chiropodist.

Insomnia

If remedies from your doctor or chemist fail, try this. Or try this first and you may not need to go to a doctor. Make sure that you have left at least one hour between the end of your final meal and preparation for bed. Get a little exercise after your meal, out of doors in the fresh air after your meal. Before getting into bed, stand and breathe deeply three times, before an open window if possible. Once in bed, and before finally settling for sleep, give yourself a moment or two quietly to let the day go. This is sleep-time not worry-time. Experiment with the best position to start sleep. Perhaps on your tummy with your head to one side. Maybe lying on your left side, with your legs curled up a little and your top arm across your body towards the under arm. Start breathing in a gentle regular pattern.

Make sure you are warm enough but not too warm. Let the air circulate through your bedroom with an opened window. In the winter in particular it's warmth *under* your body, rather than piling it on top of you that prevents you becoming cold in the night. Place a quilt or thin duvet on your mattress, then a lightweight under-blanket and then your undersheet. This way you can still sleep on a firm mattress if you prefer but the quilting underneath you gives that extra warmth and cuddliness. It will make all the difference and is far more effective and healthy than turning up the heating in an airless bedroom.

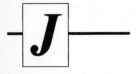

Joints that crack

A lot of people wonder if there is something wrong with them if their joints crack. Usually it is a good sign, that there is movement taking place inside a healthy joint. The surfaces of the freely movable joints, such as the knee and finger joints, are enclosed by a fluid-filled capsule. The 'pop' that you sometimes hear when the joint moves is caused by the sudden release of a bubble of gas (carbon dioxide) from the capsule of fluid. When you have treatment from an osteopath, as he releases the tensions or pressures during his manipulation of your joints, a loud cracking noise is an audible sign to you that the energies have been released.

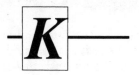

Know your limits

We all have natural limits in everything we do. Get to know your natural limits and keep within them whenever you can to avoid the sort of stress that builds up and creates on-going tension. If you have to stretch yourself beyond these limits, whether it is to do with your work, domestic life, physical abilities or emotionally, assess if you can how long this period will be for, so that you can see an end to it. It is easier to get through a demanding period if you know its probable duration before you start. If not, and of course there can be all too many occasions when situations are not in your sole control, the stress does build up. The individual nowadays is being treated more and more like a number or a machine, especially at work. If a machine is overworked it blows a fuse which is quickly and easily replaced. If you are overworked, your fuse takes longer to repair and may leave you vulnerable. Can you find your own philosophy for life, something to help you at a personal level, a religion, a group therapy, a peace-seeking yoga, or a mental attitude that supports you? Find, if necessary, and maintain your self-respect and 'proper pride' so that no one can push you around, or if they do you have learned how to detach and cope without detriment to yourself. Or, if necessary, have 'the courage of your convictions' and withdraw yourself from the situation altogether. You are the first person that has to live with yourself!

Knuckles

Don't force your rings over your finger joints. This could damage fine nerve endings or superficial blood vessels causing irreversible problems later.

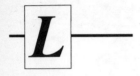

Laxatives

You must prevent constipation at all times. But only use laxatives when absolutely necessary. It is far better to improve your diet to maintain a healthy system. If you do find you need a laxative, avoid overdoing it and purging your system, especially if you are slimming. You will lose vitally necessary protein tissue which will affect your exercising performance as well, and you will also perhaps feel faint after a 'heavy trip' to the lavatory. Then you may need to eat or drink to sustain yourself, and you are supposed to be on a diet! Too strong a purgative also disturbs the sodium/potassium balance. So take care with the dose, especially to begin with, until you have got the quantity of your chosen laxative right. Herbal laxatives are kinder to your system. Two recommended to try are: Potter's 'Cleansing Herbs' and Nylax pills both available from your health store and the latter from most chemists.

Lifting

Lift heavy or cumbersome things with care. You must protect your spine. Squat down to the object if it is low, pull in your tummy muscles as you straighten up and keep the load close to you. Make sure two of you lift really heavy or awkward objects.

Alternate the hip that you carry your child on and when he really is too heavy for you don't go on lifting him. Bend down to him to comfort him, take him on your lap or cuddle him in your chair or bed. Always use the pushchair as he gets older. You are saving your back for later life. A problem started with small children doesn't always fully repair because your workload with children never stops.

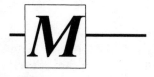

Massage

Massage is probably the oldest form of medicine because it is an instinctive treatment. If you knock against something accidentally, you rub the injured area. If your shoulders or back ache, you put your hands over the area to soothe and heal. If your child falls over you say 'Let me rub it better'. Massage is remedial: it is soft tissue treatment, assisting the circulation of blood through your body, soothing or stimulating your nervous system, helping to eliminate waste or poisonous products, increasing the action of your heart and thereby stimulating your blood supply and improving your respiratory system. It can prevent muscle wasting from injury or paralysis, and can benefit your joints if progressive immobility sets in due to such conditions as arthritis. It is very therapeutic for relieving stress and tension. One of the greatest benefits of massage is that it has none of the side effects that often accompany other forms of treatment.

If you think remedial massage would be beneficial to you, make sure that you receive treatment from a qualified practitioner. There are several reputable training centres. The Northern College of Remedial Massage and Manipulative Therapy has its headquarters at Blackpool and its graduates will have the letters LCSP after their names. The Northern College publishes its own Directory of Practitioners.

Some of the teaching hospitals in the UK still include Swedish Remedial Massage as part of the training of their physiotherapists, but physiotherapy has moved more towards the use of electro-therapy equipment, whereas the masseur relies almost solely on the skilled and sensitive use of his/her hands.

Your local library should have a list of practising masseurs in your area. Alternatively, telephone your local clinics and health centres and ask the receptionist if they have a qualified masseur or masseuse working there, although, if a woman, she may be a beauty therapist rather than a remedial therapist. Most remedial masseurs work on a self-employed basis. Look in Yellow Pages under 'Physiotherapy' or 'Massage'.

Migraine

There are many causes for the many types of migraine. Tension is a major cause. There is a wide variety of relaxation classes available these days, probably advertised in your local newspaper. A relaxation class recommended by word of mouth is often the best. Food allergies can also cause migraine so check your diet. (See also *Ingrowing toenails*.)

Moisturiser

It is never too early to start using moisturiser. If you wait for the first wrinkle or dry patch, it may be too late. There are two kinds: oil-in-water or water-in-oil. Oil-in-water creams are light and milky with oil droplets suspended in water, and are best suited to young or oily skins. Water-in-oil types are heavier and more suitable for dry or older skins. In both cases, the aim is to keep the skin's natural moisture inside the cells rather than let it evaporate, leaving a dry, papery or leathery surface. Moisturisers need not be expensive; one of the best on the market is petroleum jelly. If you massage your face with a small amount of it for one minute, then tissue off the residue before applying make-up (or going to bed), you will soon notice a difference. Or all the year round, and all over you, apply the moisturiser you use after sunbathing.

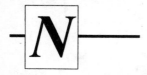

Nature

Nature is your best adviser and healer. It is most important to understand that more often than not if we would only leave the healing to nature we would get better quicker. It may mean stopping, resting, being quiet for a little while or a long while and in this hyped-up age of rushing, stress, noise and competition so many of us have obscured the gift of listening to our instincts.

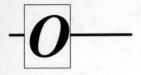

The older woman

It often is the fashion to be thin to the point of emaciation almost, even if you are older. A slender, youth-like (as opposed to youthful) face set above an 'older neck' is not everyone's idea of beauty (and we can rarely disguise ageing necks or hands). If you remove the lines and wrinkles you are removing the signs of experience and the wisdom of your maturing years, which can be beautiful to behold. Leave the laughter lines to show that you laugh! A warm heart shining through your eyes is a greater magnet than all the cosmetic 'beauty' in the world.

Other influences

Other things which affect your health and subsequently your shape are the extent to which you are happy, and the quantity of love and laughter in your life. Your ability to be positive, to maintain your individuality within all relationships, and finding and keeping occupied and stimulated, all affect your health. Smoking, drug-taking and over-eating and intemperance also have detrimental effects.

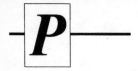

Pause

Many people, men and women, find it difficult just to stop. We get caught up in a whirlwind of pressures and demands, not least the ones we put on ourselves. It grows to be more and more difficult to take a pause in whatever we are doing or wherever we are at in our living. Much is due to our upbringing – we feel that it is almost wrong not to be doing something all the time. So many women cannot just sit and relax. They almost have to be doing something 'useful' at the same time.

We are meant to pause for rest and regeneration. If you look around you at nature, you can count so many 'pauses' that occur with rhythmic regularity throughout life. Longer-term rhythmic pauses are winter-time: the rest period after life-giving spring, growing summer and fruitful autumn; and hibernation for certain animals. The tides flow and ebb, with slack-water their pause period. Sleep is the pause and regeneration time for all creatures. Plants open and close. All this is part of the natural pattern. Human beings experience menopause, a passage of living that we need to learn to accept, cope with and welcome for the progress of our lives once we are beyond it. On a shorter scale, after each breath in and then out your body pauses almost imperceptably before the next breath in. On a larger scale, maybe 'death' is only a pause.

We need to learn to pause in our daily lives for the benefits of peacefulness, and slow down in our busy environments, that we may better cope and 'return' refreshed to our tasks.

Piles

These can be treated with anal ointment or cream and by bathing that part of you with clean, soap-free cold water. Ask at your health store for a homoeopathic or herbal remedy.

Post-natal exercises

These are essential to bring your body back to 100 per cent performance, apart from re-shaping yourself, after having a baby. Your exercises must be given to you only by your doctor, midwife or physiotherapist on an individual basis. Pelvic floor exercises (see *Urine control*) are an essential post-natal activity, to prevent involuntary incontinence.

Posture

Good posture is essential to allow your body functions to operate properly. Many of your muscles work specifically to keep you in an upright position, apart from their other functions. They work at each side and at the front and back of your body, from toe-to-top. Just standing straight, tucking in your tummy, throwing out your chest and holding up your head, as we are often instructed to do, is not necessarily producing 'good posture'. The warm-up sequence (page 88) will also tone up, strengthen and relax all your postural muscles. All curling and straightening exercises will help to re-educate your whole body and combined with relaxation in a straight line on the floor, with perhaps a pillow under your head, will help your spine to realign naturally.

Posterior

The 'bum-walk' (described on page 116) will help tone up and reduce the size of your bottom. The large gluteal muscles get a good massage as you bum-walk across the floor.

Do your best not to be too sedentary, especially at work. Exercise your hips as much as possible.

Pressure in your ears when travelling

This uncomfortable and often painful experience occurs when atmospheric pressure surrounding you changes, for example, at take-off or landing by aeroplane. If you swallow, it helps to 'pop' the pressure in your ears. This is why on an aeroplane you are often offered a boiled sweet because it is so juicy that your reaction is to swallow. Babes-in-arms, alas, cannot have this relief and their distress is considerable. By cupping your hands over their ears you create a vacuum which releases the atmospheric pressure. The moment you take away your cupped hands the pressure returns so keep your hands over their ears until you yourself are aware that the discomfort is over. Do it for yourself. It's also a good method of taking off that top level of noise at discos or concerts.

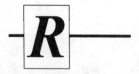

Relaxation

There are many methods of learning relaxation on offer these days, from group classes to individual work from a book. The influence may be Western or Eastern, it does not matter so long as it works for you. Eastern is the older civilisation for well-tried and recommended methods. To learn the art of relaxation, for it to be a balanced and total benefit, you need to study and practise a method which itself gives equal importance to mind and body. Mind and body cannot be divorced one from the other. Relaxation of your mind induces physical relaxation and relaxation of your body induces mental relaxation. A relaxed mind and body gives you renewed mental and physical energy to cope with the mental and physical stresses of this world. I would recommend the study of Pranayama yoga.

Roses

The gentle fragrance of roses has long been known to hold the power to relax. Many people instinctively experience this. Try walking in a garden of roses if you feel stressed or are convalescing. Rose essence, which can be bought in a bottle, is a powerful anti-depressant with antiseptic powers.

Rough hands

Put a ½ teaspoonful (2.5 ml) of sugar into the palm of your hand with an equally small amount of oil. Mix these into each other and 'wash' your hands with the mixture. The abrasive sugar grain will take away rough skin leaving the skin smooth. Any kind of oil will do: sun-tan oil, cooking oil, butter. Remember what your hands were like when you came back from holiday? A few days of sand, sun-oil and salt water makes your hands smooth very quickly. It's the same principle of abrasiveness and oil. Use it for your feet, heels and elbows.

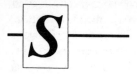

Salt

Salt is essential to life. It is found naturally in many foods and therefore is not required as an additive. If you feel you need it perhaps you should be eating more fresh or raw food, cooking in less water, cleansing your palate by cleaning your tongue daily each time you clean your teeth, drinking more water or changing your diet altogether. If you are a smoker, meat-eater or heavy drinker, your palate will have become de-sensitised and you will have lost the fine art of smell and taste. You possibly heavily over-season everything in order to experience taste and smell. A short fast or semi-fast is an excellent way to introduce change.

Salt and bicarbonate of soda

This combination in warm water has a healing and soothing effect. You can use this concoction for douching should you have congestion in your sinuses, as a gargle if you have a sore throat, and to bathe wounds. The ratio is 600 ml/1 pint water to 5 ml/1 teaspoonful of salt to a large pinch of bicarbonate of soda. The salt helps to heal and the bicarbonate of soda helps to loosen the mucus or pus.

Scout's pace or twenty-twenty

If you are trying to improve your aerobic capacity and your physical staying power through exercise, scout's pace or twenty twenty is better for you than jogging. Jogging is sustained exercise and very demanding. Scout's pace introduces its own form of pacing by the very nature of what you do. You pace yourself with alternate walking, running, walking, running. The running can be a gentle trot to begin with. Start by walking 20 footsteps and then trot or run 20 paces. Revert to an equal number of walking paces and so on. Keep the number of steps equal in both walking and running even though you will cover a much greater distance whilst running. Start and end with walking. Pacing yourself like this gives you a burst of effort followed by a more rested period.

Sedatives

Try to avoid tranquillisers if possible. Natural sedatives are watercress, lettuce, celery, chamomile tea and the smell of roses (see also *Roses*).

Shoelaces

If you have a high instep and wear lace-up shoes, do you experience discomfort over the top of your foot? The anterior tibial nerve passes down the centre of the top of your foot and pressure from lace-up shoes, especially if you use round laces, can cause considerable pain on the top of your foot and also give you pins and needles and other acute pains in or under your toes, especially the big toe and second toe. Use flat laces instead of round ones, and lace your shoes so that the criss-cross is uppermost (i.e. visible) alleviating the pressure on your foot. Fashion boots and wellingtons which are pre-moulded can cause the same problem if they fit too tightly on the top of the foot.

Sinusitis

Inflammation and sepsis in the sinuses is a distressing condition, in which the sufferer literally faces living through a blur of pain and congestion. Some of the following suggestions are worth trying:

1. Inhale hot steam, perhaps with menthol crystals. Hold your face over a steaming bowl of hot water, with a towel over your head and the bowl to concentrate the vapour. Do not use boiling water.

2. Douche, with the following recipe: to 600 ml/1 pint of warm water add 5 ml/1 teaspoon of salt and a large pinch of bicarbonate of soda. The salt is a natural cleanser and healer and the bicarbonate of soda helps to release congested phlegm and scabs from the inside of your nostrils. This flushing of your nostrils gives your sinus passages a chance to drain.

3. Sharp contrasts in temperature build up the congestion and with the congestion the pain. Try to keep an even temperature throughout your house and not have too marked a contrast between inside and outside. This can be difficult to achieve considering the excessively high temperatures that are common in modern offices and shops, especially when the outside temperature in winter is low.

4. Don't drink or eat anything that is too hot. The reaction in your mouth and sinus passages when it cools is rather like watching a bowl of hot custard cool down – it forms a skin. In other words, an impermeable and viscous congestion sets up.

5. Similarly, wash your face in water that is neither too hot nor too cold.

6. The sinus drainage apertures are high in your nostrils and when mammals evolved they walked mostly on all fours, head down, with the sinuses draining easily

in this position. Now that *homo sapiens* is vertical, our sinuses don't drain so well and man has not evolved sufficiently to rectify this problem. All upside down positions help to drain your sinuses, but you should *never* get into an inverted position if you suffer from high blood pressure or heart problems of any kind.

7. Avoid dairy products as they encourage mucus formation.

Sleep

Quality of sleep rather than quantity is desirable. We can get by on very few hours if the quality is there. Unless you are a natural 'night-bird' (in the minority) the three hours before midnight give the best rejuvenation, sleepwise. If you balance your energies equally throughout the day sleep is the ultimate participation. Settling for sleep is not the time for worrying or planning. There's nothing more you can *do*, this day. This is sleep-time. *Good* sleep is absolutely essential to promote healing and a sense of general well-being, to renew your energy and bring a sense of calm. You will be more relaxed, mentally and physically, and find you can generally cope better. It will also help you with the self-discipline required when slimming.

Smile!

Do you prefer to be greeted by a glum face or by a smile? Just watch the number of gloomy faces that pass you in the street! Does a smile cheer and lift you? This works the other way round, of course. If you smile, someone else can be on the receiving end! To smile can become a good habit. It's another form of giving. And they say that people who laugh a lot never get ulcers.

Smoking

So much has been said and written now about the dangers of smoking, and since about 1975 a gradual, successful decline in smoking has been achieved. Many of our GPs and health workers have set an excellent example.

If you are a hardened smoker you will inhale. Nearly all smokers inhale. Unfortunately all non-smokers in the company of only *one* smoker, inhale! This is called 'passive smoking'. A non-smoker wishes neither to smoke nor to inhale the poisonous toxins but alas has no choice in the company of even one smoker, perhaps in a train, restaurant, office or home. He can truly say 'I am a non-smoker but today I have "smoked" ten cigarettes'. His clothes will have absorbed the smoke and he will continue to 'inhale' long after the offender has gone and until those clothes have been washed or aired.

If you are a smoker, your taste buds and sense of smell will be less sharp. Many ex-smokers are astounded to discover that they can taste and smell again.

Sneezing

An enormous amount of energy goes into the act of sneezing, strenuously using all your muscles involved in respiration. If you are a noisy, violent sneezer it can put quite a strain on your abdominal muscles and therefore your low back. If you bend your knees a little as you sneeze (if you remember in time!) this will relieve any strain.

Standing

If you find standing for any length of time tiring, do you prop yourself up against something, or take the weight more on one leg than the other? Too much of this affects the alignment of your pelvis and spine because you will tend to use the same side all the time. Practise standing with your legs straight and your feet slightly apart to increase your base of support. This balances your body weight absolutely evenly and once you have got into the habit of it you will find you can stand for much longer before you begin to tire.

Stress

This is an ever increasing condition these days. Stress starts in your mind and then overspills into your body. Learning mentally and physically to relax is the answer. It is not wise to undertake a slimming diet or a different form of exercise if you are under stress. The extra self-discipline might be just a bit more than you need at the moment and, being human, if something has to fall by the wayside it will probably be the diet! Wait until life is more stress-free first.

Stretch marks

Pregnancy and childbirth may cause stretch marks on your thighs, hips and abdomen. Also, if you diet and lose a considerable amount of weight you may find similar markings, on your thighs in particular. Prevention is possibly the only way of coping. Be very strict about keeping your skin in these areas well lubricated with a really effective moisturiser and after each bath gently massage right round your middle with olive oil. You can try to remove stretch marks with calendula oil or vitamin E cream (apply warm) but success cannot be guaranteed.

Sun-oil

If you use sun-oil when you sunbathe, and especially if you use a 'heavy' one, make sure that you wash it all off daily with hot water. Otherwise it will clog up the pores of your skin, preventing your body from sweating and the end result may well be heat-stroke, which can make you feel giddy and disorientated.

Sunshine

It is essential to our health, development and well-being. Unfortunately in many parts of the world there is little sunshine throughout the year and during long winter months daylight hours are also at a premium. When you can enjoy sunshine with warmth and heat, you are wise to sun-tan gradually and avoid actual burning. If you are a fair-skinned, typically Nordic type with freckles you will burn more quickly and easily than if you have a darker skin. Always use a sun-screen with a filter factor to suit your skin. The fairer your skin, the higher the SPF (Sun Protection Factor) should be. Look for sun-screens with protection against both UVA and UVB rays.

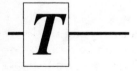

Teeth

Keep your teeth, whether they are yours or the National Health's, in good order. You need them to chew which is the first preparation of eventual digestion. Bad teeth (apart from their cosmetic appearance) can set up problems such as ulcers and the subsequent poisons may spread to your neck, as the nearest muscles into which they can drain, and if your condition is severe perhaps into your shoulders and upper back. What you are calling fibrositis may be caused by bad teeth rather than by sitting in a draught. They may also contribute to swollen neck glands and to sinusitis.

Tension

Once you actually stop, whether to relax from a hard day's work, on holiday or by withdrawing yourself from a stressful situation, the actual 'withdrawal symptoms' can be quite unpleasant. Have you ever gone on holiday and actually felt worse for the first day or two? This is tension in your system easing and can manifest as a headache or a physical ache, or just 'feeling awful'. Don't be alarmed. It's a positive sign of 'letting go' and is the forerunner of feeling better and relaxed.

Too-tight jeans

This style of trouser is still very popular but can cause three problems in particular. Firstly, the seaming that runs beneath you will press and rub against your body and in time may actually cause your skin to split. It's then very painful and you may need a specific cream. If you have washed your jeans in too-hot water and they have shrunk or if you have put on weight, and either way are squeezing yourself into them you are lining yourself up for this problem of very sore cracking. Also, as you become older, especially past menopause, your skin in this area tends to dry and thin and you are more susceptible to this problem.

Secondly, trousers that are too tight don't allow a flow of air around your thighs and private parts and combined with nylon as opposed to cotton panties, thrush might occur. (Thrush is a yeast infection, *Candida albicans*. It causes a red, itchy rash and must be treated by your doctor.)

Thirdly, if you have a sensitive low back the pressure of the very hard seams can cause low back ache. The seams are not going to give, so your body has to take the consequences.

Travelling by train, and drinking

Have you ever experienced difficulty drinking from your cup of tea or coffee when travelling on a train? If your feet are on the floor you are probably subconsciously resisting the motion of the train and the liquid tends to slop out of the cup. If you take your feet off the floor and just let them hang in space, your body will move in unison with the direction of the train and you will drink more successfully.

Typist's neck and shoulders

A long day at the typewriter or keyboard puts strain on your neck and across your shoulders. The nerves down to your busy fingers leave your spine at neck and shoulder level and your activities are reflected back to this area. You may arrive home quite stiff and sore. Try the following suggestions to alleviate this.

Exercise one

SP   Sit firmly on a chair or stool, so that you have room to swing your arms without the chairback getting in the way. Place your finger tips on your shoulders.

Keep your finger tips on your shoulders throughout, and swing your elbows down, forwards, up, back and down again in as wide a sweep as possible. Repeat 3 times.

Exercise two

Fetch a face towel and roll each end in towards the middle until the rolls meet. Secure if necessary with safety-pins or elastic bands but keep the finished roll soft and malleable. Now lie on the floor on your back and place the towel under you, longways down your spine. Bend your knees keeping your feet on the floor, turn out both hips, place your hands one on each side of your ribs and breathe in and out rhythmically for five or ten minutes. This is a very gentle way of massaging the area that is bothering you.

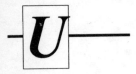

Urine control

The following exercises help to strengthen the muscles in the base of your pelvis and as you perfect the movements you will gain better control of your bladder and prevent 'leaking' when you cough or sneeze. Women who have recently had babies should do these exercises.

Exercise one

When you go to the lavatory deliberately stop and start the flow of urine. If you do this several times a day it's an excellent prevention against incontinence in later life.

Exercise two

SP Lie on the floor on your back with your knees bent up and your feet flat on the floor.

Tighten the muscles round your rectum (back passage) until you feel a squeeze and lift inside. Increase the tightening until you feel your vaginal area lift. Relax to SP. Repeat 2 or 3 times, several times a day. Do this exercise in bed if you prefer.

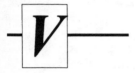

Vegetarianism

There are many reasons why people become vegetarians but I have never read or heard of it harming anyone who was previously healthy and who, as a vegetarian, maintains a balanced diet.

If your instinct indicates that you should become a vegetarian you should find the change a natural one. If you have other, external, reasons, make the change gradually as your system has to adjust to your *mental* dictate rather than to your instinctive dictate. If you need information, contact *The Vegetarian Society* at 53 Marloes Road, London W8 6LA.

A lactic vegetarian eats no meat, poultry or fish. A vegan eats no eggs or dairy produce either.

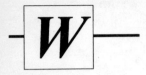

Walking

Place one foot directly in front of the other when walking. With practice this becomes automatic and can correct any minor misalignment of the spine. Your hips swing freely, your abdomen pulls in, your waist lifts, your back straightens, your shoulders relax, arms swing, your neck stretches and your head is held erect. It looks good too!

Water

Water sustains life and whereas you can survive a comparatively long time without food you can only live a few days without water. Your body is made up of about 70 per cent water and your brain consists of an even higher percentage! You need to drink water daily (at least three glasses) to cleanse and flush your system and to prevent constipation. Unfortunately, many of its natural qualities are lost because man has tampered with it, with pollution, additives and fluoridation. Pure spring water can't be beaten and its softness also benefits your skin, removing dirt and grime easily with a resulting smooth texture. If you soak your laundry overnight in soft spring water the dirt seems to drop out and a cleansing agent or detergent is often not necessary.

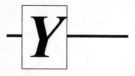

Yoga

There are over 200 different forms of yoga of which about 50 have come to the West. All were originated some 6,000 years ago. 'Yoga' is the Sanskrit word for 'unity'. The ultimate aim of all yogas is Peace of Mind. For the philosophy to be a yoga, it must also include the study and practice of detachment and breathing exercises. Most yogas have a bias, whether physical (Hatha yoga), meditative (Raja yoga), mental, mystical, medical, political, religious, etc.

Pranayama yoga is a totally balanced yoga with no bias. It is non-religious, non-political and non-competitive. This way of life teaches relaxation of the mind and body enabling the individual to eliminate mental and physical tension. This form of yoga gives the ability to face the ruthless demands of the rat-race without fatigue in mind and body. The unique sequence of breathing and physical movements are especially designed to improve concentration and circulation.

There are trained teachers of Pranayama yoga. If you are interested in knowing more about it, write to Ken Cobral, 8 Chad Road, Edgbaston, Birmingham B15 3EN, and he will give you the name of a teacher in your area.

Recommended reading

If you are interested to read in a little more depth, the following books and leaflets are worthy of your attention.

An excellent series of pamphlets and booklets are available from: Tesco Advice Centre, Tesco Stores Ltd, Delamare Road, Cheshunt, Herts, EN8 9SL. They include *Tesco Guides to Healthy Eating* and *Tesco Consumer Advisory Service Fact Sheet*.

Fasting: The Ultimate Diet by Allan Cott, MD, published by Bantam Press. This is possibly out of print but you could try in second-hand bookshops.

Food Combining for Health – Don't mix foods that fight. A new look at the Hay System by Doris Grant and Jean Joice, published by Thorsons in paperback.

Day Light Robbery – The importance of sunlight to health by Dr Damian Downing, published by Arrow Books Ltd in paperback.

Faber's Anatomical Atlas – edited by A. K. Maxwell, I. M. Burdon and S. Macdonald, published by Faber & Faber Ltd, in paperback.

The Lotus and the Rose – The art of relaxation by Yogini Sunita, available from Ken Cobral, 8 Chad Road, Edgbaston, Birmingham B15 3EN.